Routledge Revivals

Infant Welfare

Infant Welfare: For The Student & Practitioner was published in 1926, at a time that saw the development of the new Infant Welfare centres, which began to appear in the UK in the late 19th century. The book sets out the ways in which The Mother & Child Welfare Act (1918) envisaged local authorities developing ways to improve outcomes for both mothers and young children. *Infant Welfare* also provides invaluable practical detail concerning the requirements of the new Welfare centres. The aims of the centres were the maintenance of health in infants & young children, the education of mothers, treatment of minor ailments and the early detection of disease. Chodak-Gregory emphasizes the preventative nature of the work, with nurses and health visitors gaining a knowledge of the specific living conditions of individual families. She also stresses the importance of air and sunlight in a child's life, in line with the Open-Air Schools movement, which had also taken off in the early twentieth century. The centres were, for the first time, giving mothers the time and space to voice their concerns.

Infant Welfare discusses the need for positive doctor-patient and doctor-nurse relationships in order to achieve the best outcomes for mothers and children. The author's views on the doctor's workload resonate just as much today with NHS staff under enormous pressure as when the book was originally published. Fathers are absent in this book, as if they have no role in childcare, and it is the mothers who are addressed, at times in an overly prescriptive voice, reflective of the class divide at the time, but Chodak-Gregory also recognises the immense difficulties working-class women faced.

Infant Welfare reflects the growing significance of women's contribution to medicine and to wider society. There has been much written on infant welfare & working-class maternity in the late 19th and early 20th centuries in the past few decades. Chodak-Gregory's *Infant Welfare* is an important document by a pioneering female doctor. It bears witness to the commitment of the doctors, nurses and voluntary workers involved and to the working-class women, who attended the Infant Welfare centres, bringing the materiality of their lives into close focus.

Infant Welfare

For the Student and Practitioner

Hazel H. Chodak-Gregory.

With a new introduction by Gill Gregory

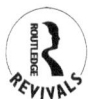

Routledge
Taylor & Francis Group

First published in 1926 by H.K. Lewis & Co. Ltd

This edition first published in 2026 by Routledge
4 Park Square, Milton Park, Abingdon, Oxon, OX14 4RN
and by Routledge, 605 Third Avenue, New York, NY 10158.

Routledge is an imprint of the Taylor & Francis Group, an informa business

ISBN 13: 978-1-041-09078-6 (hbk)
ISBN 13: 978-1-003-64834-5 (ebk)
ISBN 13: 978-1-041-09079-3 (pbk)
Book DOI 10.4324/9781003648345

REISSUE OF *INFANT WELFARE* BY DR. HAZEL CHODAK GREGORY

Acknowledgements

I would like to thank the following friends, colleagues and organisations who have helped me along the way in this project – Isobel Armstrong, Nicola Bion, Betty Bradbury, The British Society for the History of Paediatrics & Child Health, Sarah Broady, Morwenna Chaffe, Mary Cuthbert, Rhian Davies, Harriett Gilbert, Lesley Hall at The Wellcome Library, Christopher Hilton, Helena Hilton, Dr Anthony Hulse, Mari Joyce, Sally Kilmister, Bella Millett, Leonee & Richard Ormond, Harriet Parks, Victoria Rea, The Royal College of Paediatrics & Child Health, The Royal College of Physicians, UNISON, Lynne Walker at the Institute of Historical Research (University of London) & The Wellcome Collection.

Especial thanks to Frances Parkes, my editor at Routledge, for her enthusiasm, encouragement and professionalism.

Many thanks, as ever, to my family for their love & support over the years.

Gill Gregory, London, 19th May 2025.

CONTENTS

1 Dr Chodak Gregory, 'Physiognomy of Disease in Childhood', Presidential Address to the Medical Society, May 18th, 1931, 109, Vol XXVI, July 1931, *Magazine of the London (Royal Free Hospital) School of Medicine for Women.*

TIMELINE

Dr Hazel Chodak-Gregory (née Cuthbert), 1886 – 1952

1904	Hazel Cuthbert, aged 18, enrols at the London (Royal Free Hospital) School of Medicine for Women.
1911	Qualifies in medicine, M.B., B.S.
1915	M.R.C.P.
1916	Appointed Medical Registrar, Royal Free Hospital.
1917	Marriage to Dr Alexis Chodak-Gregory.
1920	Birth of Basil Chodak-Gregory.
1922	Dr Hazel Chodak-Gregory in post at Royal Free Hospital until **1951** as Assistant Physician, Senior Physician & Consulting Physician for Children's Diseases.
1926	Hazel H. Chodak Gregory, ***Infant Welfare***, published.
1932	Vice-Dean, London (Royal Free Hospital) School of Medicine for Women.
1934	2nd woman to be elected a Fellow of the Royal College of Physicians (F.R.C.P.) by her male peers.
1939–1945	Dean, Three Counties Emergency Hospital, Arlesey, Bedfordshire – Royal Free Hospital base branch for the duration of World War Two.
1945–1951	Physician & Consulting Physician for Children's Diseases, Royal Free Hospital.
1952	Death on 12th January, aged 65.

NEW PREFACE TO THE REISSUE OF *INFANT WELFARE*

It is remarkable to consider that nearly a century has passed since Dr Hazel Chodak Gregory's pioneering book, *Infant Welfare*, was published in 1926, and the relevance it has for modern times. Paired with a fascinating Introduction by her grand-daughter, Dr Gill Gregory, describing her extraordinary grand-mother, her family and their connections, for example, with the composer, Benjamin Britten, this book gives a fascinating insight into one of the for-midable female pioneers in medicine, most notably in Paediatrics and Child Health.

Clearly much has changed in 100 years – then there was no childhood obesity epidemic, nor the extensive programme of immunisations that we have today, but the underlying philosophy, 'prevention is better than a cure', a concept much repeated by politicians today, was a relatively new concept at that time. *Infant Welfare* sets out in detail what this meant in practice with remarkable insight, along with the challenges that preventative child health work faces. 'Preven-tative work is less cut-and-dried than curative work', Chodak Gregory writes, and yet today this vital work is the first in line for cuts when there are financial challenges.

Infant Welfare combines practical advice on communication with mothers with scientific detail on the composition of various milks, the required accom-modation arrangements for an Infant Welfare clinic and the various Acts of Parliament which provided the necessary framework for Infant Welfare work. Chodak Gregory's opinions are expressed confidently and unambiguously. That confidence and ambition is seen in the description of her grandmother by Gill Gregory, but we also see a woman who came across as quite shy and reticent. She clearly had a strong and intriguing personality, which can be seen clearly in the photographs of her included in this very welcome new edition.

Like most doctors at that time she would have had extensive experience of treating sick children – what is now called Paediatrics – yet chose to write this book on preventative medicine – what is now called Child Health. Specialisa-tion, especially in children's medicine, was in its infancy in 1926. It took another 70 years, in 1996, for the new Royal College to combine those concepts to

become the Royal College of Paediatrics and Child Health after much contro-
versy and debate. Dr Hazel Chodak Gregory was way ahead of her time.

This is a book that should appeal to a wide audience, including those interested in the struggle still faced by women in male dominated professions in the
21st century, the history of the development of medicine and its relationship to
the social sciences and particularly those interested in the history of Paediatrics
and Child Health.

Dr Anthony Hulse, MD, FRCPCH

President, British Society for the History of Paediatrics and Child Health

June 2025

DEDICATION

In memory of my grandmother, Hazel H. Chodak-Gregory
1886 – 1952

NEW INTRODUCTION TO THE 2025 REISSUE OF *INFANT WELFARE*

June 9th 2011

I had arrived in the large entrance lobby of UNISON[2], the trade union head-quarters on the Euston Road in London, and I was looking through a glass wall, separating the steel-framed office block (within which I stood) from the warm red brick of a Victorian building, incorporated within the new structure. The old building was originally The New Hospital for Women, founded in 1872 as a hospital run exclusively by women, by the pioneering doctor, Elizabeth Garrett Anderson (1836 – 1917), who was the first woman to be appointed as a visiting physician at the East London Hospital for Children in 1870. She went on to co-found the London School of Medicine for Women in 1874, where she would become Dean in 1883.[3]

From the other side of the glass wall, I saw a party in full swing, many guests having gathered to celebrate the opening of the Elizabeth Garrett Anderson Gallery, a permanent exhibition recording the history of women in medi-cine. I stood in the present, looking into the past and its celebration. Having stepped inside, I joined in the applause as a huge cake was carried in. Dave Prentis, the General Secretary of UNISON at the time, gave a speech on the long history of women's struggle for equality and paid tribute to the women doctors who figure in the exhibition. He also acknowledged all the women involved – the nurses, midwives, ancillary workers and others - in addition to the more well-known pioneers. He thanked Dr Lynne Walker of the Institute of Historical Research (based at the University of London) and others who had been involved in mounting this wonderful exhibition, to which I had contrib-uted some materials relating to my grandmother, Dr Hazel Chodak-Gregory. Dr Lesley Hall, a member of the curatorial team and an archivist at The Wellcome

---

2 Trade union for public sector employees.
3 Garrett-Anderson refused to allow her name to be used while she was alive, but following her death in 1917, the New Hospital for Women was renamed the Elizabeth Garrett Anderson Hos-pital in her honour.

Library, would help me greatly in my subsequent research of my grandmother's career at the Wellcome.

My friend and colleague, Leonee Ormond (Professor Emerita of Victorian literature at King's College, London), arrived and, wine glasses in hand, we walked into the exhibition rooms, adjacent to the party space. Much of the display was made up of graphic and electronic exhibits. Pioneering women were projected onto the walls. The stories of doctors, nurses and midwives were told, some for the first time.

Guests circled a large interactive screen and then I saw my grandmother's image swimming on the surface toward me. Her dark hair was up in an elegant roll and she was smiling, her blue eyes gently lit – 'Dr Hazel Chodak-Gregory (née Cuthbert) (1886 – 1952)'. The photograph was taken when she was in her late twenties[4] and Leonee turned to me, smiling, 'Your grandmother was beautiful.' I was very glad to be related to such an impressive pioneer but sad that I had never known her as she died several months before I was born in 1952.

In March, 2025, I was invited by Dr Anthony Hulse[5], a senior consultant paediatrician who established the Department of Diabetes & Endocrinology at the Evelina London Children's Hospital[6], to give a lecture on my grandmother's life and career at the annual conference of the Royal College of Paediatrics & Child Health, which met later in March at the SEC Armadillo, one of the conference buildings that comprise the Scottish Exhibition & Conference Centre on the north bank of the Clyde in Glasgow.[7]

My lecture, *Dr Hazel Chodak-Gregory: pioneering paediatrician,* was scheduled in between presentations on the history of rickets (which my grandmother discusses in *Infant Welfare*) and the history of NHS paediatrics in Glasgow.

---

4 The photograph of Dr Hazel Gregory, Fellow of the Royal College of Physicians (FRCP), is held at the Heritage Centre, Royal College of Physicians, 11 St Andrews Place, NW1 4LE. Copyright held by Dr Gill Gregory.

5 Dr Hulse is also the President of the British Society for the History of Paediatrics & Child Health (BSHPCH).

6 The Evelina London Children's Hospital was founded in 1869 in Southwark Bridge Road, south London. It was named after Evelina Gertrude de Rothschild (1839 – 1866), the wife of Baron Ferdinand de Rothschild, who died, with her child, in premature labour. The hospital came under the management of Guy's Hospital in 1947 and became part of the NHS in 1948. In 1976 the Evelina Hospital closed and the children's wards moved to the newly built Guy's Tower. In 1999 the hospital was re-established as a new specialist hospital for all children's services at Guy's & St Thomas' in Lambeth.

7 The SEC Armadillo, a name given it by Glaswegians owing to its armadillo-like scales, opened in 1997. Norman Foster, the architect, had in mind the interlocking series of ships' hulls to be seen on the Clyde.

A lecturer in English Literature, I found myself among a host of pae-diatricians, which felt strange but, in some sense, familiar. My father, Dr Basil Gregory – Hazel's son – was a consultant psychiatrist and, when I was a child, I did meet some of his friends and colleagues, including child psychiatrists. One of them had a delightful way of squatting down so he could talk with me at eye level. As a non-scientific person I am finding this 'new' world of paediatrics fascinating.

Dr Hazel Chodak-Gregory (1886 – 1952)

Hazel (as I shall call my grandmother) died on the 12th January 1952, five months before I was born in the June of that year. My mother was into her second trimester and visibly pregnant, when she and my father attended Hazel's funeral in a light and airy chapel at Golders Green crematorium, which was packed beneath its high gabled rafters with Hazel's family and friends, colleagues and former patients.

The tributes that appeared in the many obituaries not long after my grand-mother's death were lengthy. The *British Medical Journal* (2nd February 1952) writes of her 'outstanding' career in paediatrics, stating that she took a wide view of the medical care of children, 'realizing that it involved a knowledge of social and preventive medicine as well as clinical skill and experience.' Hazel's focus on social and preventive medicine was shared by many paediatricians at this period and in *Infant Welfare* she sets out the key features of preventive medicine and how to put them into practice at the Infant Welfare centres.

The obituary notes her appointment as 'acting assistant physician, at the Royal Free Hospital' in 1916, during the First World War (1914 – 1918), an ap-pointment that was confirmed three years later when she 'became assistant phy-sician'. In 1927, 'when the children's work was separated from general medicine and the Riddell wards for children were opened at the Royal Free', she would become children's physician to the hospital.

During the Second World War (1939 – 1945), she was posted to the Three Counties Emergency Hospital (a base branch of the Royal Free during the war) at Arlesey in Bedfordshire, where 'she was acting dean for the duration' as the resident physician in charge, with care of the children's wards and the general medical beds. 'In 1935,' the obituary continues, 'she became the second woman to be elected a Fellow of the Royal College of Physicians' by her male peers, which was a rare distinction. The first woman to be elected was Dr Helen Mackay (1891 – 1965).

The *BMJ* obituary quotes some of my grandmother's colleagues. 'O.R. & G.B' write:

> Dr Gregory was always a stimulating teacher and had the great gift of expecting the best from everyone. At the same time, she had a tolerant outlook and a strong sense of values, which enabled her to overlook the shortcomings of others. [...]

It was at Arlesey [during the Second World War] that she became so well-known and loved by all with whom she worked. She made an outstanding success of this difficult appointment, integrating the work as a whole and organizing with enthusiasm the social as well as the clinical side of the hospital. She was naturally shy and reserved, and this at times made her appear somewhat unapproachable, but those who came to know her and to be admitted to her friendship realized her great charm, her integrity, and her unselfish readiness to help others. Throughout her life she accepted difficulties with philosophy and courage, especially when she faced so magnificently the losing battle with ill-health.

'F.G.' writes: 'Those of us who were residents at Arlesey will always remember the evenings spent with her in friendly and stimulating discussion, and we shall always be grateful for her encouragement and wise counsels.'[8]

The distinguished paediatrician, Dr Bernard Valman[9], kindly sent me the British Paediatric Association obituary, which refers to Hazel working 'quietly and unostentatiously' whilst 'gaining recognition as perhaps the foremost woman clinician in London [...] She was for a long time Chairman of the Medical Committee of the Royal Free Hospital.' Hazel's shyness is again mentioned but at Arlesey, the reviewer writes, 'her light could no longer be hid [...] she established herself in a unique position, admired and trusted by all, a beloved figure who did not fail them in times of difficulty and hardship.'[10]

In *The Lancet* 'J.D. McL' writes,

The peaceful happy wards in her control reflected her own calm happy personality. During the war her work was transferred to the E.M.S. Hospital[11] at Arlesey, and her old beautiful wards in the Gray's Inn Road [Royal Free Hospital] were destroyed by a flying bomb; but no commotion or disaster could overthrow the serenity of her mind. All her friends – and they were all who knew her – wished her the many peaceful years of retirement which she had so well earned but did not live to enjoy.[12]

The *Royal College of Physicians* obituary notes that in 1919 the Royal Free Hospital appointed her as the hospital's 'first woman physician'.[13] Dr Beryl D. Corner,

8 278, Feb. 2, 1952, Vol 1, 1952 January to June, Obituary, *British Medical Journal*, BMA London.
9 Dr Bernard Valman is the author of *BMA Children's Symptoms*, Dorling Kindersley, 1997.
10 H.C. Cameron, *The British Paediatric Association 1928-1952*, BPA, 1955.
11 The Emergency Medical Service was established during the Second World War (1939-1945). It was a state-run network of free hospital services organised by the Ministry of Health. The EMS is often credited as being a forerunner of the National Health Service (NHS) established in 1948.
12 218, Jan 26 1952, Volume One January-June 1952, The *Lancet*.
13 'Hazel Haward Chodak-Gregory', 71, Vol V, *Royal College of Physicians*. The word 'consultant' was not used prior to the NHS (1948). All senior doctors in hospitals were known as 'Honoraries'

in a letter to myself (2006), wrote of my grandmother being 'the first woman to be an honorary physician at any London teaching hospital following her graduation [in 1911] during World War I.' She said she remembered my grandmother from when she was her student at the London (Royal Free Hospital) School of Medicine for Women between 1928 and 1934. 'All medical students spent one month attached to the Children's Department [at the Royal Free] and were taught by your grandmother at that time.'[14] Una C. Ledingham[15], a female physician, who knew my grandmother very well, provides more personal history in her obituary,

[…] Hazel Cuthbert came second in a family of six, born and brought up in an atmosphere predominantly literary and artistic. In that home kindness and consideration prevailed, and, though discipline was exerted, punishment and threat were alike unknown. Thus a happy background contributed to the development of natural gifts.

From early on, when little more than a child, her expressed ambition was to qualify and to practise medicine. Family funds were low, but her unswerving determination led an uncle to back her – a decision he never had cause to regret.

An outstanding student career fully justified the faith in her intellectual and practical abilities, for neither then nor later, when tackling the higher examinations, was she to know academic failure.

After qualification her progress continued […] The apparent ease with which she gained the necessary experience is a measure of her excellence, at that time when substantial opposition to the place of women in the profession was widespread. In 1926 as Assistant Physician, to both the Royal Free Hospital and Shadwell Children's Hospital [now the Queen Elizabeth Hospital for Children] her position was assured. At this time, by ill-fortune, the two Senior Physicians of the Hospital [Royal Free] retired together, leaving Hazel Gregory, as she had by then become, to step up into the position of Senior Physician, at the early age of 40. At the same time the new Children's Department had recently been completed, and was literally waiting for her to assume command. After much weighing

---

as they worked in a voluntary capacity without any payment. Doctors working at local authority hospitals were usually paid and full-time.

14 Beryl Corner, OBE, FRCP (1910 – 2007) was a paediatrician, who pioneered neonatology – care of the newborn, especially premature babies.

15 Una Christina Ledingham (1900 – 1965), a British physician known for her studies of diabetes in pregnancy, trained at the London (Royal Free Hospital) School of Medicine for Women and was awarded an MD London (1927) & FRCP London (1947). She was a member of the Board of Governors, Royal Free Hospital (1957-1960).

of the points at issue, and what must have been deep heart searching, she turned her back on the glamour and status of the Senior Physicianship, reconciling herself to abandon her interest in general medicine, and side stepped to become the first head of the Children's Department, feeling that here lay her prime duty. From then on she identified herself completely with her new work, without any expressed regrets for what she had given up in the old, and by her energy, enthusiasm, and example, founded a department second to none in the general teaching hospitals in London.

In 1935 she was elected the second woman Fellow of the Royal College of Physicians, but with the outbreak of war, and the chaos created by the evacuation her life was again disturbed. The Royal Free Hospital base branch was situated 40 miles out at Arlesey, at that time a bleak and unfriendly place [...] the content with which residents settled there, the continuity established for visiting staff, and the building up of a little cultured oasis in the middle of the stark fields, lay to her credit.

[...] In appearance she was somewhat awe-inspiring, of striking height, with an aloof, almost austere dignity, and a deep blue penetrating, often disconcerting gaze. She had no small talk, and no use for such, being singularly unconcerned by trivialities. She was neither small minded nor self-seeking, yet her sense of humour was well developed, and she had a knowledge of human nature and a depth of affection not always realised.

Never intruding, nor proffering unasked opinion, her clear- sighted judgment and sympathetic advice were ever at the disposal of those in need.

To work for her was an enviable experience, and once she trusted that trust was complete, she neither interfered nor questioned. Indeed she had a happy knack of explaining away another's mistakes as though they were inevitable, while allowing any success to rank as personal achievement. The fortunate ones, having once been selected to work for her, were backed to the hilt, and she was not satisfied until she had set them on the pathway to success. Not a few of her colleagues owe their present position to her efforts. We shall miss her sadly.[16]

Before my father, Dr Basil Gregory's death in 1990[17] I had only seen a couple of photographs of Hazel, which were taken at my parents' marriage in the summer

---

16 18-19, 'Obituary: Hazel H. Chodak Gregory, M.D. B.S., F.R.C.P. (*née* CUTHBERT)', Vol XIV, 1952, *The Royal Free Journal.*

17 Dr Basil Gregory (1920 – 1990) was the first Director of the Paddington Day Hospital (St Mary's Hospital) in the 1960s, an experiment in group psychoanalytic therapy, continuing the work of Dr Wilfred Bion & others with traumatised soldiers during the Second World War (1939 – 1945).

of 1949, when she was sixty-three. In those she appears as a dignified and graceful woman.

The few photographs my father left give some impression of how her life had unfolded. The first is a studio photograph of her family of eight – her parents, three sisters, two brothers and Hazel herself. The family look typically Edwardian, with the women and girls wearing high neck dresses, with trim frills, and the men and boys in blazers. The father, Goymour Cuthbert (1849 - 1902), is wearing a light summer suit and a boater, looking rather like the writer, H.G. Wells[18].

Hazel is sitting next to her father, an earnest looking child of about fifteen years old. Her hair is tightly scraped back and hanging loose down her back. Her father, Goymour, was the youngest of five sons of a Suffolk squire and over six feet tall. He was an architect of renown, designing the Royal Courts of Justice restaurant in the Strand, 'the handsomest and most elegant bar bank in London'[19], described as 'a shining example of Victorian architecture at the peak of the Victorian age' with 'electric light […] and air conditioning.'[20] Sadly Goymour died only a year or so after the family photograph was taken. He 'suddenly fell down dead from heart failure in 1902' at the young age of fifty-three[21], when Hazel was sixteen years old.

In the photograph father and daughter share a similar expression of seriousness and intensity, even though Goymour is sporting a boater. In another photograph Hazel is in her mid-twenties and wearing a graduation gown, with long pointed sleeves, along with the graduation doctors' velvet bonnet, with golden tassel. Having graduated in 1911, she is looking pleased with her achievement, but not ecstatic. Two photos of Hazel were taken toward the end of her life. In the first she is wearing a white doctor's coat, with a stethoscope tucked into the pocket. Now in her sixties Hazel looks drained and ill. She is suffering from arterial sclerosis and will die soon. In spite of her serious illness there is still good humour and warmth in her eyes. In the remaining photo, taken at about this

---

My father was a full-time consultant for the NHS as well as in training as a psychoanalyst in the 1960s. There is a small holding of his papers, P42, at the Institute of Psychoanalysis archive, created by myself.

18 H.G. Wells (1866 – 1946), author of *The Time Machine* (1895), *The War of the Worlds* (1898) and many other novels, short stories, political treatises and works of science fiction. Many New Women (or feminists), of the late 19th & early 20th centuries, appear in his novels.

19 *Penny Illustrated Paper*. See 'Our History', *Outer Temple Chambers* website.

20 Despite its sumptuous interior the restaurant closed after 3 years and was, in 1895, converted into the well-known Lloyds Bank, 222-225, the Strand ('Our History', *Outer Temple Chambers* website). Goymour Cuthbert also designed Cornhill House (1896) & Drapers' Hall, both with sculptures by Herbert Pegram (1862 – 1937).

21 Michael Gilbert, Volume 15, *Contemporary Authors Autobiography Series*, 1992.

time, she has aged greatly, but looks less stressed. She is playing with some puppies, cocker spaniels, and is laying on the grass, surely making the most of the time she has left. She died on the 12th January 1952 at the early age of sixty-five. There is a plaque at the Royal Free, paying tribute to her eminent career, alongside plaques to other women pioneers [22] in medicine.

Hazel was born on 20th July, 1886, at 15, Portsea Place in London, not far from the Kensington Gardens in Hyde Park, where in 1912 George Frampton's iconic bronze sculpture of Peter Pan would appear as if by magic overnight, to the delight of the children who visited the next morning on the 1st May – Mayday.[23] There were other addresses for the family. Hazel's nephew, Michael Gilbert (a celebrated writer of detective fiction), writes of the family living 'in an old-fashioned house in Harewood Square', a beautiful Georgian square in Marylebone, where the main line station now stands. The upper middle-class family, he writes, lived 'a happy and comfortable life, from which anything sordid or dramatic was as rigorously excluded as the draughts from a day nursery.'[24]

In the family photograph Hazel's mother, Marion Linford (1857 – 1941), is standing, with her hands resting on the shoulders of her son, Olaf, who sadly died in action in 1916, on the Somme, aged twenty-six. She looks like a strong, capable woman. Marion's grandson, Michael Gilbert, describes her as 'a woman of spirit'[25]

One of Marion's nephews was Sir Maurice Linford Gwyer, a lawyer who became Chief Justice of India (1937-1943) and was one of the founders of Miranda House[26] (the founder Principal being Veda Thakurdas[27]), a red brick college for women at the University of Delhi, in 1948, which is today one of the top ranked colleges in India. In a photograph taken after the Oxford University

---

22 Elizabeth Garrett Anderson (1836 – 1917), Sophia Jex-Blake (1840 – 1912), Isabel Thorne (1834 – 1910) & others.

23 George Frampton was commissioned by the author, J.M. Barrie, to make the sculpture, which was erected overnight and appeared in Kensington Gardens on May Day, 1912, so that children might believe that the fairies had placed it there overnight. In 1929 J.M. Barrie gifted his copyright of *Peter Pan* to Great Ormond Street Hospital (GOSH), a hospital for children in Bloomsbury, London. Barrie jokingly said that 'at one time Peter Pan was an invalid in the Hospital... and it was he who put me up to the little thing I did.' In 1988 The House of Lords granted the hospital the right to a royalty from *Peter Pan* in perpetuity.

24 Ibid, Gilbert.

25 Ibid, Gilbert.

26 One of the reasons Sir Maurice gave for choosing the name 'Miranda' for the college was that she appears in Shakespeare's *The Tempest*.

27 Veda Thakurdas was the first woman to attain an MA from Punjab University in 1930 and a Tripos from Cambridge. Under her leadership Miranda House won international recognition as a premier institution of higher education for women. In 1920 the London (Royal Free) School of Medicine for Women, with the co-operation of the India Office, opened a hostel for Indian women medical students.

Convocation on 7th August 1940, Sir Maurice is pictured next to the Nobel prize-winning poet and philosopher, Rabindranath Tagore (1861 – 1941), who had just been awarded an Honorary Doctorate by Oxford University. Sir Maurice bears an uncanny and striking resemblance to my father, Dr Basil Gregory, and also to Hazel. He lived in Eastbourne, Sussex and he may have been the uncle who funded Hazel's studies at the London (RFH) School of Medicine for Women. On her application form the Testimonial is given by a teacher at Rippingale school in Eastbourne, who had known Hazel for 'the last five years'.[28] Sir Maurice's sister, niece of Marion Linford, was Barbara Gwyer (1881-1974), the Principal of St Hugh's college, Oxford (1924-1946), where she taught the late Barbara Castle, the Labour Party Employment minister.[29] Strong, high-achieving women were clearly a feature of my grandmother's family.

Hazel was the second of six siblings, four girls and two boys. Her brother, Milroy Cuthbert (1889 – 1970) became a vicar and her younger sister, Berwyn Cuthbert (1888 – 1970) – who married Bernard Gilbert, the Lincolnshire poet[30] – trained for a year as a nurse at the Evelina Hospital for Sick Children in London before being appointed Superintendent of a newly founded Infant Welfare centre in South Lambeth in 1916. In 1923 she began to work for Glaxo, the company producing dried-milk baby food (Glaxo is from the Latin *lacto*, meaning milk), using the excess milk produced on dairy farms. The product was sold with the slogan 'Glaxo builds bonnie babies'.

Berwyn worked first in the advisory service, lecturing visiting nurses, who were studying the research work at Glaxo, before being assigned the task 'of selling Glaxo and its increasing nutritional products, to infant welfare clinics and public health authorities.'[31] Soon after the Second World War broke out in 1939 she was appointed Woman Power Officer to one of the Ministry of Labour Manpower Boards, where her knowledge of the problems of married women in industry proved invaluable. On her retirement in 1948 she became the full-time mothercraft editor of the *Housewife* journal, writing 'scores of major articles on mothercraft topics' and answering 'literally thousands of letters from her readers. She spoke frequently on women's programmes on BBC radio and lectured all around England.[32] She also wrote several books on childcare, including *The Housewife Baby Book* (1948), *Love & Laughter: philosophies of motherhood* (1954) and

28 Dr Gill Gregory, family archive.
29 Barbara Castle backed the women sewing machinists at Fords in 1968, which led to the Equal Pay Act in 1970. The dispute and Barbara Castle's key role were memorialised in the award-winning film, *Made In Dagenham* (2010).
30 1882–1927. Gilbert's poetry evokes rural life in Lincolnshire. He also wrote about the Home Guard during the First World War.
31 'Death of Mrs. B.M. Gilbert', *Glaxo Group News*, March 1970.
32 Ibid, Glaxo.

Seven to Seventeen: on child welfare (1959), all of which she wrote under the name of 'Anne Cuthbert'.

> Hers was a full life, lived to the full for others. An ardent feminist, a pioneer of infant welfare and an authority on mothercraft, Mrs Gilbert will be long remembered with affection and admiration...and will assuredly endure through her Anne Cuthbert books.[33]

In later life Hazel and Berwyn shared a flat at Makepeace Mansions, on the Holly Lodge Estate in Highgate, for a short period when, prior to the 1950 General Election (won by the Labour Party, with a much-reduced majority), two posters were seen in their window – Hazel's Conservative Party poster and Berwyn's Labour Party poster. Makepeace Mansions are tall, Tudor-style mansion blocks, referred to in the neighbourhood as the 'Tudor cliffs'. The blocks had been built by The Lady Workers' Homes Limited, the association having been founded in the 1920s to provide accommodation for 'the educated woman of small means'. [34]

By 1950 Hazel had very limited funds following the bankruptcy of her husband, Dr Alexis Chodak-Gregory, in 1949, when Alexis also revealed that he had been keeping a second family in the wings for over ten years without Hazel's or my father, Basil's knowledge. Berwyn's poet husband, Bernard Gilbert, had abandoned her with four small children at the outbreak of the First World War, when he went to work for the Ministry of Munitions, never to return. Apart from a small legacy she was then dependent on her earnings.[35] The two sisters, despite being abandoned by their respective husbands, were nonetheless impressive and formidable in their achievements. They are inspiring forebears.

Berwyn and Bernard's son, Michael Gilbert (1912 - 2006), the writer of detective fiction, was also a solicitor, who numbered among his clients Raymond Chandler, the American writer of 'hard-boiled' detective fiction. Michael's daughter, Harriett Gilbert, is a writer and broadcaster and the long-time presenter of *A Good Read* on BBC Radio 4.[36]

---

33 Ibid, Glaxo.

34 The Lady Workers' Homes Limited built the mansion blocks in the 1920s and Camden Council took them over in the 1960s.

35 Michael Gilbert, in his *Contemporary Authors Autobiography* (ibid Gilbert) writes of his father, Bernard, as 'an amiable, if distant, figure' who was 'entirely self-educated', and of his extensive knowledge of a rural district of Lincolnshire. His writing included poetry, short stories, novels and plays. Gilbert writes of his father being 'clever, single-minded and charming. He was also completely, almost pathologically, selfish.' Berwyn, though, 'appreciated his point of view. She would go her way; he would go his.'

36 I am indebted to Harriett, who has filled in many gaps in my research.

My second cousin, Helena Hilton[37], recently retired from her position as an archivist at The Children's Society in London and her husband, Dr Christopher Hilton, is Head of Archive & Library at Britten Pears Arts. He is based at the Red House in Aldeburgh, the former home of the composer, Benjamin Britten (1913 – 1976) and his colleague and lover, Peter Pears (1910 – 1986). Hazel and my grandfather, Alexis, were friends of Britten in the 1940s, when Alexis assisted in preparations for the first Aldeburgh Festival on the Suffolk coast, in 1948, where he exhibited some of his large collection of paintings by John Constable, which were sold at Sotheby's, the auctioneers, on his bankruptcy in 1949.[38]

There is a vein of Scottish blood in the Cuthbert line. In DNA tests my brother, Robert Gregory and I have discovered that we are 7% Scottish and a cousin in Hazel's family, the late Elizabeth Cuthbert, a royal archivist at Windsor, conducted research that suggests the Cuthberts are descended from 'the Family of Cuthbert of Castlehill in the County of Inverness'. The name 'Cuthbert' is Pict and signifies 'skill' (Cuth) and 'illustrious' (Bert).

In 1904 Hazel, aged eighteen, took up her place at The London (RFH) School of Medicine for Women in London and there she would live up to the 'Cuthbert' family name. Her London lodgings were at '52, Thrale Rd., Streatham', a long, broad and very straight road in south-west London. Given her family were very literary, she may well have known of the Hester Thrale connection with Dr Samuel Johnson.[39]

The London School of Medicine for Women in Hunter Street, Bloomsbury, was founded in 1874 by a group of pioneering female physicians, who included Elizabeth Garrett Anderson (1836 – 1917), Sophia Jex-Blake (1840 – 1912), Elizabeth Blackwell (1821 – 1910) and Thomas Henry Huxley (1825 –1895), the Darwinian scientist and grandfather of Aldous Huxley (1894 – 1963), a writer

---

37 Helena & Chris Hilton have helped me at every turn in my research of Hazel's family and at the Red House in Aldeburgh.

38 The centrepiece of my grandfather's collection was *The Marine Parade & Old Chain Pier, Brighton*, one of John Constable's 'six footers' in oils. The painting was acquired by the Tate Gallery in 1950, after the collection was sold at Sotheby's in 1949. See my book, *The Studio*, Free Association Books, 2016, for details.

39 Thrale Road, a street of suburban villas, is named after Hester Thrale (1741 – 1821) and her husband, Henry Thrale (1724 – 1781), who built a Georgian mansion in Streatham Park, SW London. Hester was well-known for her literary and musical salon and for her early feminism. She was also the friend and mistress of Dr Samuel Johnson (1709 – 1784) and, when her husband died, it was assumed she would marry Johnson but she was in love with her children's music teacher, Gabriel Mario Piozzi. They married and lived in Italy and Johnson died five months later. (Adam Gopnik, 'Man of Fetters: Dr Johnson & Mrs Thrale', *The New Yorker*, 8.12.2008).

much admired by Hazel's son, Basil, and many other students at Cambridge in the 1930s and 1940s.[40]

Garrett Anderson became the Dean of the new London School of Medicine for Women where, over fifty years later Hazel would be appointed Vice-Dean in 1932. Having been refused entry to multiple medical schools, Elizabeth Garrett Anderson qualified with the Society of Apothecaries in Britain in 1865, after which the Society amended its regulations to prevent any other women obtaining a licence to practise medicine. In 1876 a new Medical Act permitted British medical authorities to license all qualified applicants, whatever their gender. Garrett Anderson went on to train at the University of Sorbonne and graduated with a medical degree in 1870. In the same year she was appointed a visiting physician at the East London Hospital For Children (later the Queen Elizabeth Hospital for Children), where Hazel practised early on in her medical career.

The East London Hospital had opened in 1868 in a converted warehouse at Ratcliff Cross and in his essay, 'A Small Star In The East' (1868), Charles Dickens writes of 'the children's hospital established in an old sail-loft or storehouse, of the roughest nature […]' and of 'a gentleman and lady' having 'quietly settled themselves in it as its medical officers and directors.'[41] The couple were Dr Nathaniel Heckford and his wife, Sarah (née Goff), who had met during the cholera epidemic of 1866 and were resolved to provide medical care for children living in poverty.

Garrett Anderson[42] had founded St Mary's Dispensary in Seymour Place in Marylebone in 1866 and the Dispensary developed into the New Hospital for Women in 1872, its purpose being to give medical attention, by qualified female practitioners, to women living in poverty. The hospital moved to new premises on the Euston Road in 1889 and it was renamed the Elizabeth Garrett Anderson Hospital in 1918 after her death in 1917.

The Royal Free Hospital, founded on the Gray's Inn Road, Holborn, by the surgeon, William Marsden in 1828, was the first teaching hospital in London to

---

40 I inherited Aldous Huxley's essays, *Music at Night* (1931), from my father, Basil. The volume originally belonged to Hazel and at the end of one essay she has written in pencil, 'Go To Bed', concerned perhaps that her 12-year-old son was becoming too engrossed in ideas of consciousness. My father became a medically & psychoanalytically trained psychiatrist, and I have also inherited his 24-volume edition of Sigmund Freud's complete works, published by the Hogarth Press, 1953-1974.

41 Charles Dickens, 'A Small Star In The East' (1868), *The Uncommercial Traveller* (1875).

42 Elizabeth Garrett Anderson was also active in the movement for female suffrage, her sister, Millicent Garrett Fawcett, becoming a leading light. Elizabeth became mayor of Aldeburgh on the Suffolk coast, where she gave speeches in support of the suffrage. Garrett Anderson died in 1917 so she did not live to see female suffrage, for women over 30, being granted in 1918. It was not until 1928 that women were given equal suffrage, at the age of 21, with men.

admit women for training and in 1877 students at the London School of Medicine for Women began to complete their clinical studies at the hospital. By the time Hazel began her studies in 1904 the London School had been re-named The London (Royal Free Hospital) School of Medicine for Women.

The Royal Free, as its name suggests, had been founded as a hospital providing 'free' treatment for the poor and destitute. Its first name was 'The Free Hospital' and, on Queen Victoria's accession to the throne in 1837, it was renamed 'The Royal Free Hospital'. Children, though, until the mid-nineteenth century, were treated alongside adults in hospitals, with girls on the women's wards and boys on the men's. The first children's hospital in the UK was Great Ormond Street Hospital for Children, founded in 1852, but it did not treat babies and infants.

The Romantic movement of the late 18th and early 19th century had brought the figure of the child into close focus and in 1855 the writer, Anna Jameson, in an essay titled 'A Revelation of Childhood', asks,

> What do we know of child-nature, child-life? […] child-life we treat as if it were no mystery whatever, just so much material placed in our hands to be fashioned to a certain form according to our will and prejudices.[43]

Jameson is referring to the pervasive influence of Utilitarian theories being practised at this period, for example in schools, which Charles Dickens satirizes in his novel, *Hard Times* (1854), in which the siblings, Louisa and Tom Gradgrind, are stunted in their emotional growth and well-being, owing to their father's strict utilitarian education, whereby imaginative literature is excluded from the curriculum in favour of strictly useful 'facts'. At the same time social commentators, such as the journalist, Henry Mayhew (1812 - 1887), were interviewing homeless children on the streets of London and exposing the cruelty and neglect at the heart of the Victorian metropolis.[44]

One of Mayhew's interviews was with 'The Little Watercress Girl', who was 'only eight years of age, had entirely lost all childish ways, and was, indeed, in thoughts and manner, a woman.' The girl is unaware of the London parks ' "The parks! […] where are they?"' The child only knows the streets where she sells her bunches of watercress. She wears 'a thin cotton gown, with a threadbare shawl wrapped round her shoulders' and shuffles along in 'the large carpet slippers that served her for shoes', which might 'slip off her feet'. In her short life she

---

43 Mrs Jameson, *A Commonplace Book of Thoughts, Memories, and Fancies*, London, 1855.
44 Henry Mayhew, *London Labour & London Poor*, appeared in serial form in the *Morning Chronicle* in the 1840s and in three volumes (a triple decker) in 1851.

has taken care 'of a baby for my aunt' and helps her mother, 'who was in the fur trade'. She does have 'a box of toys' at home in Clerkenwell and 'knows a good many games' but she does not play with the toys or play games. The children on the streets, she says, do not play because they're 'thinking of our living'. Child-life itself was under severe threat on the London streets.[45]

The fictional counterpart of the little watercress girl is 'the figure of Mignon', a child acrobat who appears in the German writer, Johann Wolfgang von Goethe's *Wilhelm Meister's Apprenticeship* (1795)[46]. Mignon is an Italian child of about twelve or thirteen – 'No one has counted,' Mignon replies, when asked her age. She belongs to a travelling band of rope-dancers and is subject to violent spasms and fits. She dies when she sees her older friend, Wilhelm, making love to an adult woman.[47] Mignon's growth is stunted and she dies without seeing womanhood, which was the fate of many street children in London at this period. Girls sometimes became child prostitutes and had babies, which were invariably abandoned on the streets or drowned in the Thames.

A growing awareness of the appalling suffering of children on the streets coincided with the birth of Paediatrics as a separate and distinct discipline, which was still in its infancy when Hazel applied for admission to The London (RFH) School of Medicine for Women in 1904. The British Paediatric Association (BPA) – the first of its kind – was not established until 1928. The first president was George Frederic Still (1868 – 1941), a physician and paediatrician from a working-class background, who won a scholarship to Cambridge University and went on to identify what is today known as 'Still's disease', a form of childhood arthritis. He also established the department of childhood diseases at Guy's Hospital in 1893.

A history of the BPA states,

> During the first 17 years of its existence the BPA was an entirely male preserve [...] a club for gentlemen interested in Paediatrics.
>
> [...] In 1944 a momentous decision was taken to elect women after a postal vote in which 34 were in favour and 12 against. No time was lost and in 1945, Dr Catherine Chisholm [...] was made an Honorary member and Drs Helen Mackay [...], Hazel Chodak-Gregory [...] and Beryl Corner [...] ordinary members.[48]

---

45 'The little watercress girl', Vol. 1 (1851), ibid, Mayhew, *London Labour & London Poor.*

46 *Wilhelm Meisters Lehrjahre* (1795) was translated by Thomas Carlyle in 1827.

47 Mignon is the central motif of Gill Gregory's 'Past Children, Past Selves', review of Carolyn Steedman's *Strange Dislocations. Childhood & the Idea of Human Interiority 1780 – 1930*, 1995, in No 2, Vol 8, *Women: a cultural review* (1997), Oxford University Press.

48 Forfar, Jackson & Laurance, *The British Paediatric Association 1928 – 1988,* BPA, 1989.

In 1996 the Royal College of Paediatrics & Child Health became the successor to the BPA. The addition of 'Child Health' draws attention to the importance of preventive medicine and a more wide-ranging approach, a significance that was the hallmark of the practices and theories of the early women pioneers in medicine, such as Hazel Chodak-Gregory.[49]

By the time female doctors were admitted to the British Paediatric Association in 1945 Hazel had practised as a paediatrician for over 30 years and had been distinguished as only the second woman to be elected, in 1934, a Fellow of the Royal College of Physicians (FRCP). This was eleven years before women were admitted as members of the BPA.

In 'Pride, prejudice, and paediatrics (women paediatricians in England before 1950)'[50] Dr David Stevens has written that 'allowing a woman to become a fellow of the Royal College of Physicians and gain entry into the inner sanctums of a 400 year old male monopoly was a moment of symbolic importance.' The decision to allow women to be elected to fellowship was made in 1924, despite the opposition of the registrar of the college [...] who complained that 'women were not up to it [...]'.[51]

Stevens writes of the campaign for women to enter the professions beginning in the 19th century. In an earlier book[52] I discussed the work of the Langham Place Circle, an association of women established in 1858, whose offices, reading room & coffee shop were at 19, Langham Place in central London, where *The English Woman's Journal* (1858 – 1864) was published. In 1859 the Society for Promoting the Employment of Women was established with a training and job register for 'ladies who wish to become candidates for remunerative employment in charitable institutions, as nurses in hospitals, matrons in workhouses, teachers or superintendents in industrial schools [...] [53].

The Langham Place Circle women visited factories, hospitals and schools, where they recorded the work and conditions of the women employees. The circle was part of a wider movement for social and political change which gathered momentum in the late 19th century. Amy Levy (1861 – 1889) in her essay,

---

49 In March, 2025, at the annual conference of the RCPCH, I met many paediatricians, who are keen to introduce their students to the history of paediatrics and how that history can inform and illuminate paediatrics practice today, at a time when the NHS (founded in 1948) is under such severe stress.

50 David Stevens, 'Pride, prejudice, and paediatrics: women paediatricians in England before 1950', 91: 866-870, *Archives of Disease in Childhood*, 2006, BMJ Publishing Group Ltd & RCPCH.

51 Ibid Stevens.

52 Gill Gregory, *The Life & Work of Adelaide Procter: poetry, feminism & fathers*, Ashgate/Routledge, 1998/2019.

53 Extract from a circular printed by the Langham Place Circle in 1860.

'Women & Club Life' (1888)[54], sets out the many restrictions ambitious women of the period faced,

> In class-room and lecture-theatre and art-school, college and club-house alike, woman is waking up to a sense of the hundred and one possibilities of social intercourse; possibilities which, save in exceptional instances, have hitherto for her been restricted to the narrowest of grooves.

David Stevens writes,

> The early women doctors of the 19th century who were forced to obtain their training on the continent – in Zurich, Bern and Paris – were part of a political movement and transatlantic network concerned with issues of women's rights, universal suffrage, women's health and public health measures. These women who 'stormed the citadel' wanted to, and did, change society as well as medicine. Opposition to women's entry into medicine was led by doctors who defended the male monopoly against the threat to their prestige [...] They argued [...] women's bodies, intellect, and temperament were not up to the demands of studying medicine, let alone practising as doctors. These arguments did not stop, but echoed down the 20th century long after women had gained the right to qualify in medicine.[55]

Stevens continues, 'Well into the 1930s, advertisements for many of the posts in the *British Medical Association* stated that only men could apply.'

Hazel qualified in medicine in 1911, just a few years before the First World War began in 1914. 'Both wars [First & Second World Wars] allowed women to advance in the professions and in medicine. The London medical schools opened up to women medical students in the First World War, only to bar them again [...] after the end of hostilities [...] by 1930 University College Hospital [...] was the only co-educational London Medical School.'[56]

Stevens states that 'few of these women [paediatricians] were married; the path for a woman paediatrician with a family was very difficult. Hazel Chodak-Gregory, who had a wealthy sympathetic husband, was the only one

---

54 Amy Levy, 'Women & Club Life', June 1888, *The Woman's World*.
55 Ibid Stevens.
56 Ibid Stevens. The Royal Free Hospital had admitted women into training in 1877 but as part of the London School of Medicine for Women, which had been renamed The London (Royal Free Hospital) School of Medicine for Women in 1896.

of these women paediatricians who married and had a family.'[57] Alexis, with his many contacts in London's social, cultural and medical circles, may have facilitated her remaining in post after their marriage at Hampstead St John church on the 17th December 1917.

My grandfather, Dr Alexis Chodak-Gregory's favourite painter, John Constable, lay buried in the churchyard of St John's – the quintessentially English painter he was perhaps fighting for on the battlefields of the Somme, where he was awarded the Military Cross in 1916, having applied for (naturalization) and become a British subject, which secured his eligibility to fight for his adoptive country.

Her wartime romance and marriage to Alexis would find Hazel at the heart of the cultural zeitgeist in Bloomsbury, where she and Alexis lived in Russell Square. Figures such as Virginia and Leonard Woolf were neighbours in Tavistock Square. Virginia Woolf (1882 – 1941) was only four years older than Hazel and her novel, *Mrs Dalloway*, was published in 1925, just a year before Hazel's *Infant Welfare* appeared in 1926. In the novel Elizabeth Dalloway, Clarissa and Richard Dalloway's daughter, walks out of the doors of her home in Westminster – her father is a Member of Parliament – onto the streets of central London, 'It was so nice to be out of doors [...] out in the air'. She takes an omnibus and finds herself 'rushing up Whitehall' and onto the Strand, wondering what her future might hold,

[...] she might be a doctor. She might be a farmer. Animals are often ill [...] she would like to have a profession [...] possibly go into Parliament...[58]

Hazel was the 'new'[59] kind of woman Elizabeth Dalloway was imagining. Such women appear in Woolf's friend, E.M. Forster's novel, *Howard's End*, published in 1910, a year before my grandmother graduated in 1911, in the form of Margaret and Helen Schlegel, upper middle-class sisters living in central London, 'They talked to each other and to other people [...] They even attended public meetings. In their own fashion they cared deeply about politics, though not as politicians would have us care; they desired that public life should mirror whatever is good in the life within. Temperance, tolerance and sexual equality were intelligible cries to them.'[60]

57 Ibid Stevens. Stevens provides descriptions of the Women Fellows of the Royal College of Physicians (1934-53).

58 147-150, Virginia Woolf, *Mrs Dalloway* (1925), Penguin, 2000.

59 The New Woman was to be seen in reality and in fiction at this period. She was satirised, often viciously, in newspapers & journals as a manly, cigar-smoking woman, who rode bicycles and wore loose fitting clothes rather than stays or corsets. She supports various campaigns, including the suffrage.

60 E.M. Forster, *Howard's End* (1910).

Dr Alexis Chodak-Gregory, a Jewish-Russian emigré from Tashkent, welcomed the advent of the New Woman. He had lost his entire family (who were murdered in Tashkent, according to him) when he arrived in Glasgow, Scotland, at the age of sixteen or seventeen and, like so many refugees, he put the past behind him and reinvented himself in his adoptive country. In marrying Hazel he became part of the central London zeitgeist and embraced the 'new' world of modernity, emerging after the First World War. He and Hazel must have made an impressive and striking couple – he was short and Hazel tall – as they strolled, more likely hurried, around Bloomsbury like figures in a Futurist[61] painting.

Before meeting Alexis, Hazel's progress in her medical career had been rapid. The Royal Free record of her achievements is impressive. Having qualified in medicine in 1911 at the age of twenty-five, she went on to become resident Surgical and Medical officer at the Birmingham & Midlands Hospital for Sick Children.[62] In 1914 Hazel was appointed as Assistant to Clinical Pathology at her parent hospital, the Royal Free, and in the August of the same year, when the First World War broke out, she was recruited by Dr Louisa Garrett Anderson (1873-1943)[63] and Dr Flora Murray (1869-1923) to the Women's Hospital Corps (WHC), a surgical unit comprised of women doctors and trained nurses, which was to report to the French Red Cross in Paris.

The stylishness associated with Paris was to be seen in the uniform of the Corps, which consisted of a skirt, several inches shorter than the usual ankle-length skirt, with a loose, buttoned tunic of a greenish-grey colour. Small cloth hats with veils and overcoats to match 'made a very comfortable and useful outfit […] Parisians murmured, 'C'est chic, ça!' […] Feminine, graceful, business-like, it was invaluable as an introduction to the character of the Corps.'[64]

In Paris the WHC were based at the Hôtel Claridge, 'a large modern caravanserai on the Champs Élysées', which became a hospital for the treatment of sick and wounded soldiers. The hotel had been built in 1914, and it was not yet open when it was requisitioned by the Ministry of Armaments for the duration

---

61 Futurism was a movement of artists & writers originating in Italy in the early 20th century, which celebrated dynamism, speed, technology, cars & aeroplanes, along with cities & the machinery of cities.

62 The Birmingham Children's Hospital today. The hospital was founded in 1862 by Thomas Pretious Heslop (1823 – 1885), a social reformer, philanthropist, physician & Professor of Physiology at Queen's College, Birmingham. Heslop was also the author of 'The Realities of Medical Attendance on the Sick Children of the Poor In Large Towns', Royal College of Physicians, Edinburgh (1869).

63 Louisa was the daughter of Elizabeth Garrett Anderson.

64 10-11, Part 1, Ch I, Flora Murray, *Women As Army Surgeons* (1920), 2024.

of the war when, in 1918, at the conclusion of the conflict, the doors officially opened.[65]

The War Office in the UK were not interested in recruiting women doctors, which was why the WHC were based at a French hospital, organised by the French Red Cross. French journalists were astonished to find women surgeons and often asked, 'Who is it really who operates?'

One editor, to whom the surgeons were indicated in person, contemplated with serious attention Dr Cuthbert [Hazel], who was young and pleasing, and then said to her:

'Et vous, mademoiselle, vouz coupez aussi?'

'Oui, je coupe,'she replied slowly; for her facility with the knife was greater than with the French tongue.

'Incroyable!' he gasped.[66]

In October 1914 a photograph was taken of surgery taking place in an operating room staffed by the Women's Hospital Corps at Hôtel Claridge. A wounded soldier is being given chloroform before being operated on by British women surgeons. Dr Flora Murray, the Surgeon-in-Charge, is administering the chloroform, assisted by Dr Marjorie Blandy, and Hazel stands to Dr Murray's left, concentrating on the procedure.[67]

Hazel was still at Hôtel Claridge that Christmas of 1914[68] and on Christmas Eve 'Red Riding Hood, a Pantomime', was staged. Hazel and Baroness Geysa de Braunecker, a Hungarian expatriate, produced an abridged version of the fairytale – 'or threw it together, for the construction left much to be desired.'

The hall became uproarious over the flight of the grandmother pursued by the wolf, and many hands were stretched out to catch the wolf and give the old lady a chance [...] The men said that they had never known such

---

65 Celebrities such as Marlene Dietrich (film actress), Edith Piaf (singer), Georges Simenon (writer & creator of the Maigret series of detective stories) & many others were known to frequent Hôtel Claridge.

66 35, Ch V, ibid, Flora Murray.

67 'The Women's Hospital Corps During the First World War', HU90880, 14.10.1914, Imperial War Museum.

68 At Christmas in 1914 there was an unofficial 'truce', when many French, German & British soldiers crossed 'no man's land' between the trenches to exchange greetings, talk, have a smoke and sing carols. Subsequently officers gave orders that there was to be no fraternization between soldiers.

a Christmas: it was something to tell in the trenches, something to write home.[69]

In 1915 the WHC relocated to the Endell Street Military Hospital, established by Dr Flora Murray and Dr Louisa Garrett Anderson in May 1915, in the former St Giles Union Workhouse building in Covent Garden, where 'all round lay the teeming, crowded streets of Soho and Drury Lane.'[70] Convoys of injured soldiers arrived daily in large numbers, having been transported from London's main railway stations, which were within easy reach.

In the face of continued opposition from the British male military establishment, the women succeeded in their work, with many commentators attributing their success to the more home-like environment they established, along with the women's ability to consider the patients' psychological as well as their physical health. The hospital adopted the motto 'Deeds not words', the same motto as that of the Women's Social & Political Union, the suffragette organisation, which from 1914 ceased their campaigning to engage in the war effort.

Hazel, having returned to London, continued her work at the Royal Free and in 1916, the year she met Alexis, she was appointed Medical Registrar. She was also Assistant Physician at the Women's Hospital for Children on the Harrow Road in west London, which Louisa Garrett Anderson and Flora Murray had established in 1912 to provide healthcare for local working class children.[71] Hazel worked at the Women's Hospital for five years and by 1918 she was also working as a tutor at the London (Royal Free Hospital) School of Medicine for Women, where she had trained.

As she had met and married Alexis during the war it is possible that they may have first met at the Royal Free after he had returned wounded from the Somme. My late maternal grandmother, Ruth Craven (née Ashwin), married my late grandfather, Eric Craven, after nursing him on the front line in France. All the men he led were killed but he survived, his shoulder blown off.[72]

Dr Alexis Chodak-Gregory (1889 – 1964) had fled his homeland, according to one source, during or after one of the two Russian revolutions in 1905. The first and most well-known revolution led to the massacre of peaceful demonstrators in the square in front of the Winter Palace in St Petersburg on Sunday 9th January that year – known as 'Bloody Sunday' – after which Tsar Nicholas II was persuaded to attempt the establishment of a constitutional monarchy. By

---

69 Ch 10, Part I, ibid, Murray.
70 Ch I, Part II, ibid, Murray.
71 'Lost Hospitals of London' website.
72 My late grandfather, Eric's missing shoulder intrigued me as a child.

the end of 1905 the second revolution occurred in Moscow where the uprising, led by Vladimir Ilych Lenin (1870 – 1924), took place between the 7th & 18th December, when an armed rebellion against the imperial government was brutally suppressed.

Accounts of my grandfather, Alexis's origins, are varied. It was the educationist and translator, Willa Muir (1890 - 1970), the wife of the poet, Edwin Muir (1887 - 1959), who located him in Moscow, in 1905, in her memoir,

> One of my friends [...] was a Russian, Alexis Gregorievitch Chodak, who had fled Moscow in 1905 after the rising in which he had been involved as a student. In the course of getting a medical degree, before going on to London, he had turned up at St Andrews University [in Scotland] and became attached to my circle of close friends. Alexis was a small, well-built man, spontaneous, attractive and very charming. He married one of his tutors [Hazel], a distinguished and delightful woman; they set up a joint practice in Bloomsbury not far from Guildford St, and Alexis became Dr Chodak Gregory, an easier name for British tongues to get round. When Edwin and I were laid low by the so-called Spanish influenza that was sweeping through London [1918-1919], I sent an S.O.S. to Alexis, who saved both our lives, as we felt at the time.
>
> [...Alexis said] we must go into the country to finish our convalescence [...] and it was nonsense for us to say we could not afford it, since it would cost us nothing. He would himself send us to a hotel he knew of in Crowborough, and all we had to do was to go [...][73]

The joint practice Alexis and Hazel set up was at 16, Gordon Mansions in Bloomsbury, near Great Ormond Street Hospital, the children's hospital established in 1852. Alexis's generosity was a hallmark of his life. He had arrived in Glasgow, aged sixteen or seventeen, on his own after his entire family had been massacred and somehow he had either brought a lot of money or had a family legacy sent to him from Russia. The following is the account my mother, Dinah Gregory (née Craven) related from when I was small.

As my father never spoke Alexis, I had only my mother's account to go on. She conveyed very few facts, the gist of which were,

> Your grandfather escaped by train from Tashkent after all his family were killed and he arrived in Glasgow. Then he trained as a doctor and worked in London. His patients called him a 'miracle doctor!' He became a very well-known doctor and had many well-known friends, including the great

composer, Benjamin Britten, and he bought lots of paintings by John Constable, but then he suddenly went bankrupt and escaped the country with his second family – his mistress, Marjorie, and one little boy and a little girl about to be born. Your father and grandmother, Hazel, knew nothing about this other family, and Alexis disappeared for a year or two. Then he was arrested in France and went to Brixton prison, but after a few months, lots of famous people went to the court to say he was a very good doctor & a very generous man, so he was released from prison! He was a great man and everyone loved him!

I found my mother's story, which she related often, compelling but confusing in that, if I so much as mentioned Alexis to my father, he looked very angry and told me nothing. My mother also conveyed the idea that 'going bankrupt' and having 'a second family' were rather glamorous attributes, involving adventures and being chased by the police. Much later in my life I began to research my grandfather's history so far as I could.

Forty years before the 1905 revolution, the Russian Imperial Army had taken just two days to defeat the defenders of Tashkent in 1865, and the Russian officials went on to Europeanize the city[74], 'with wide Petersburg-style boulevards replacing the narrow, winding, and dark alleyways and mud huts of 'Asian Tashkent' […].' Tsarist officials, though, reported that, contrary to the idea of establishing a more 'civilized' city, Tashkent Russians were 'educating Central Asians in the practices of extortion, corruption, vice, and greed', belying the supposed cultural superiority of Russian values. The colonized Central Asians, whilst resisting Tsarist authority, were highly successful in trade and dominated the marketplace. They were also practised in the art of healing and often treated local diseases more successfully than Russian doctors.[75]

A friend of my father mentioned that Alexis was known for his 'faith healing', which he accompanied with singing the folk songs of his homeland, whilst treating his patients in London, and in Brixton prison he apparently continued this practice, proving to be very popular with his fellow inmates! Hazel's nephew, Michael Gilbert, writes of his 'Uncle Alexis' establishing 'a practical monopoly in the treatment (then in its infancy) of rheumatoid arthritis […].[76] Alexis had trained at The Institute of Massage & Medical Gymnastics[77] in Bloomsbury,

74 Jeff Sahadeo, *Russian Colonial Society in Tashkent, 1865-1923*, Indiana University Press, 2007.

75 Ibid, Sahadeo.

76 Ibid, Gilbert.

77 At the first annual dinner of The Chartered Society of Massage & Medical Gymnastics at the Café Royal in Regent Street, London, R.C. Elmslie in his speech stated that 'Massage is […] almost as ancient as medicine itself' but that 'medical gymnastics' were only one hundred years old, dating from the time when Lin (Pehr Henrik Ling) founded his school in Stockholm in

which was pioneering a new Swedish treatment, anticipating many of the techniques used in massage and osteopathy today.

At the age of nine years old, in 1961, I accompanied my father on a visit to the London flat, where Alexis lived with his second family after being released from prison in 1952. In January 1952 he had appeared in handcuffs, between two prison warders, at my grandmother's funeral at Golders Green crematorium. My father, Basil, did not acknowledge him. In 1949, on returning from his post-war military service, as the only doctor at a medical unit near the Suez Canal, he had been full of enthusiasm and at the beginning of his medical career, only to find his father on the brink of bankruptcy, as well as hearing, for the first time, the shocking news of the second family he and Hazel knew nothing of up until then.

Hazel and Alexis had by then moved from Bloomsbury, where the family of three had lived at 14, Russell Square, to a sumptuous apartment at 46 Portland Place[78] (near the BBC building) not far from Oxford Circus. The actor, Ralph Richardson[79], who lived at 88, Portland Place, was a neighbour and became a friend. He, Alexis and Hazel shared a passion for flying aeroplanes, which were still an exciting new invention. In an undated letter 'Ralph' writes,

Dearest Hazel & Alexis,

Thank you so much for your kind letter and invitation. I should have answered before but have been very busy and have not been well either. I had some vaccinations and they made me feel awful [...] I am off tomorrow for Sudan to finish a film, shall not be able, unhappily, to come and hear the music. [...] John Longden was playing in the film, 'Q Planes'[80] which I have just finished and asked after you [...].[81]

all love to you both Ralph

1813. He also remarked that many in the medical profession were still unaware of the treatment. Women made up most of the membership of the Society.

78 Portland Place is the residence of John Buchan's Richard Hannay, the swashbuckling hero of the novel, *The Thirty-Nine Steps* (1915), and Portland Place appears as a location near the beginning of Alfred Hitchcock's film adaptation in 1935.

79 Ralph Richardson (1902-1983) was a Shakespearian actor who, with John Gielgud & Laurence Olivier, dominated the British stage at this period. He also appeared in numerous films, including *Dr Zhivago*, directed by David Lean in 1965.

80 *Q Planes*, Dir: Tim Whelan & Arthur B. Woods (1939) with Laurence Olivier & Ralph Richardson, a comedy/pre-war spy story. The 1960s tv series, *The Avengers*, was influenced by Richardson's portrayal of a spy.

81 Dr Gill Gregory, family archive.

In another letter from Ralph the actor describes crashing a small aeroplane in a field in Dorset. My grandparents were both early members of the London Aeroplane Club, founded in 1925 at Stag Lane Aerodrome in Edgware. Flying as a means of private transport had only recently taken off and one of my grandmother's ambitions was to fly solo, like Amy Johnson (1903 – 1941), from London to Australia but in a faster time.

My mother related that, after Alexis's bankruptcy and the abandonment of his family, 'your grandfather and your father had a fist fight on the doorstep of their home in Portland Place and Dad knocked your grandfather to the ground.' My father had broken with Alexis immediately and the visit my father and I made, in 1961, was an attempt at a reconciliation. They had not met for ten years, and Alexis had by then had several minor strokes.

My memory of that day is still vivid. I was entranced by my sturdy little grandfather, who was about five foot two. He kept patting my head and chuckling and then danced with me around the sitting-room. Some kind of reconciliation was effected. I remember Alexis looking rather ashamed and my father seeming tentative, if very moved by the meeting. My grandfather also sang folk songs every so often during our visit. He was very charming.[82]

Alexis and Hazel met in 1916 in London, either in a medical setting or at friends. The story goes that, he being short and Hazel tall, he had gazed up at her and fallen in love with 'the beautiful doctor' at first sight. The year before, in 1915, Alexis had a brief and passionate affair with the Welsh composer, Morfydd Owen (1891-1918), who went on to marry Ernest Jones (1879-1958), the psychoanalyst and Sigmund Freud's official biographer. Morfydd Owen's biographer, Dr Rhian Davies [83], has recently discovered that during the time Alexis was at St Andrew's University and meeting members of the Russian circle, such as Willa Muir, he was also teaching elementary and advanced Russian, and folklore, at various technical colleges and institutes in Dundee, Arbroath and Perth. His classes were advertised in the *Dundee Evening Telegraph*, the *Dundee Courier* and the *Arbroath Herald & Advertiser* in July and September, 1916. Alexis is described as 'a native of Taratoff [Saratov], in south-east Russia' and as a graduate of Petrograd [St Petersburg] University, 'currently studying medicine at Dundee University College.' The *Arbroath Herald* reports that 'over fifty gathered to welcome Mr. Alexis Chodak' and after treating 'his large class to a most

---

82 See my book, *The Sound of Turquoise*, KUP, 2009/10 (autobiographical fiction) for an account of my 'folk hero' grandfather, and also my art memoir, *The Studio* (Free Association Books, 2016) for a discussion of some of his paintings by John Constable and my grandfather's involvement, with Benjamin Britten, in the first Aldeburgh Festival in 1948.

83 Rhian Davies, *Yr Eneth Ddisglair Annwyl/ Never So Pure A Sight: Morfydd Owen (1891-1918)*, Gomer Press, Wales, 1994.

interesting two hours' instruction in Russian phonetics [...] the enrolments in the class have been so numerous that it will be found necessary to divide it into two'.[84]

The DNA tests my brother Robert and I had revealed that we are not Russian at all but a quarter Jewish and if Saratov, a city in south-west Russia, is where Alexis had his origins, then his family may well have been killed in a pogrom, after which many Jews fled east as well as west, which would explain the story of his fleeing Tashkent.

Despite his bankruptcy and desertion of Hazel and Basil in 1949, Alexis had been very supportive of Hazel's medical career throughout, as David Stevens has pointed out. In the early 1920s Hazel worked as an Assistant Physician at the Royal Free and continued as an Assistant Physician at the Women's Hospital for Children in the Harrow Road. She also practised at The East London Hospital For Children founded by Dr Nathaniel Heckford (1842 - 1871) in 1868, which moved to Glamis Road, Shadwell, in 1877.[85]

1926 saw Hazel at the peak of her career when she was appointed Physician for Children's Diseases at the Royal Free. She had also become a mother by then. My father, Basil, Alexis and Hazel's only child, had been born on December 6th, 1920, when Hazel was thirty-four years old. In a photograph of Hazel holding her small child, he is pulling away from her, looking toward the photographer, Alexis perhaps. Her eyes are lit up with joy and tenderness.

The photograph reminds me of William Rothenstein's painting, *Mother & Child* (1903)[86], in which his wife, Alice Rothenstein (née Knewstub), holds up her small son, John, who is gazing toward the window in their high-ceilinged sitting-room in Hampstead. Hazel, in the photograph, and Alice, in the picture, are both wearing loose dresses with open necks, their hair up in rolls and swept off their faces, looking every inch the modern, forward-looking women of the period.

In 1926, her annus mirabilis, Hazel's book *Infant Welfare: For the Student and Practitioner*[87], was published, the year the new Children's Department was established at the Royal Free.

When the Riddell[88] Wards for Children, were officially opened at the Royal Free early in 1927, Queen Mary of Teck[89] presided. The wards were supplied

---

84 *Arbroath Herald & Advertiser for the Montrose Burghs*, 22.9.1916.

85 The hospital closed in 1963.

86 Tate Britain.

87 Hazel H. Chodak Gregory, H.K. Lewis & Co. Ltd., London, 1926.

88 George Riddell, 1st Baron Riddell (1865 – 1934), newspaper proprietor & representative of the British press barons at the Paris Peace Conference (1919-1920), contributed over half the £50,000 raised to build the children's wards. Riddell was the President of the Royal Free Hospital. My grandmother was presented to Queen Mary of Teck at the opening.

89 George V's Queen consort.

with 20 cots for boys up to the age of 10 and 20 for girls up to the age of 12. An open-air sun terrace gave the children access to fresh air, a feature of the Open Air Schools movement, which had been gathering momentum after the First World War. The movement began in Indiana where the 'sunlight treatment', along with fresh air, good ventilation and nutritious food, were heralded as a new approach to treating children with tuberculosis and malnutrition, whilst providing them with an education. Hazel and Alexis were both advocates of Open Air Schools.[90]

My father (Basil), aged six, attended the Regent's Park Open Air school, between 1927 and 1928. The school had been established in 1913 in the Botanical Gardens for the Royal Botanical Society's subscribers, the school's objective being to provide pupils with 'the best of physical health combined with a sound and rational education.' Children aged four to twelve years old were accepted and the charge was £5 to 9 guineas per term depending on the age of the child. The classes were held only in the mornings between 9.15 and 12.30 and the children sat at small desks beneath the trees, weather permitting. If there was inclement weather the classes were held in the Fellows Room, a large colonial-style ballroom with verandas.[91]

The Institute of Massage & Medical Gymnastics in Bloomsbury – where Alexis trained – advocated exercises and 'drill' in the open air.[92] Alexis was passionate about the importance of good physical health and he seems to have been a very robust man. He may, at some stage, have grown up on a dacha with farmland and he went on to farm his own land very successfully in Huntingdonshire in the 1930s and 1940s. His service, during the First World War, as a lieutenant in the Royal Army Medical Corps, who tended to his men on the field of battle at the Somme, won him a Military Cross for bravery, suggesting that he was physically fit and strong.

Basil flourished at the Open Air school in Regent's Park, attaining high marks and many '1st in class' assessments. But he does not excel in 'Rhythmic Exercises & Drill' and is described in reports as 'somewhat detached and shy'. Alexis, by all accounts, was not shy whilst Hazel is described as shy and reserved in many of the obituaries. Like mother, like son, perhaps.

90 In 1914 the sisters, Rachel and Margaret Macmillan, organised an open air school in the garden of Evelyn House, Deptford. By 1937 there were 96 open air days schools in Britain.

91 See 'Lost Hospitals of London' online website for details of the Regent's Park Open Air School.

92 Massage and Medical Gymnastics became more institutionalized in Europe and North America from the late 19th century, especially in London and Paris, and the practice of physiotherapy was also increasing, with the incorporation of physiotherapy departments in several hospitals. See Gregory Quin, 'The Rise of Massage & Medical Gymnastics in London and Paris before the First World War', 1-24, 34(1), *Canadian Bulletin of Medical History*.

By 1932, when my father was twelve, he was a boarder at his Prep school, St Peter's, on the Sussex coast, and in that year Hazel was appointed Vice-Dean of the London (RFH) School of Medicine for Women. In 1935 she was elected a Fellow of the Royal College of Physicians (FRCP) and in the same year Hazel and Alexis bought *Houghton Grange* in Huntingdonshire (now Cambridgeshire). The Grange was a large country mansion set in a 39-acre estate and Hazel was the official owner so it is possible that Alexis was already running into money troubles.

Even though he continued to practise in London on a much smaller scale, Alexis now also owned three farms, which were adjacent to *Houghton Grange*. He worked long hours on the farms, tending a prize herd of Ayrshire cattle[93] and paying the best farm workers and cattlemen, from all over the country, way over the odds. Hazel and Alexis, being passionate about the benefits of a healthy life, planned to develop a Treatment Centre and health farm at the Grange for people living in poverty. In a newspaper report of his arrest in France after the bankruptcy[94] and flight from the country in 1949, Alexis is quoted as saying, 'I had dreams that I would make enough money to give my services in medicine free to the poor – but my health broke down. I had been gassed during the First World War.'[95]

By this time Hazel and Alexis had become friends with Benjamin Britten (1913 – 1976), probably after the war but perhaps earlier, and in 1946 Britten gave Alexis the score of *Peter Grimes* (1946), with a handwritten dedication, 'alas, no Constable, but the best I can do!'[96] He also gave Alexis the scores of the operas, *The Rape of Lucretia* (1946) and *Albert Herring* (1947), both with hand-written dedications. The dedication to *Albert Herring* is signed, 'with my best wishes and thanks for [your] great help for the first Aldeburgh Festival.'[97] In his dedication, referring to Constable, Britten is recognising Alexis's love of the Suffolk painter, John Constable's work, seen in his collection of over a hundred paintings, sketches and drawings by Constable, sold at Sothebys in 1949. In 1948 Alexis exhibited a selection of these works – landscapes, seascapes and

---

93 He is said to have sold a bull to the writer, J.B. Priestley (1894 – 1984), a prolific writer, most widely known for his play, *An Inspector Calls* (1945).

94 My grandfather's bankruptcy was officially recorded in February, 1950, after he and his second family had fled the country late in November, 1949, to disappear for over a year, various sightings of them being reported on the Mediterranean, in South Africa and even in South America. His debts were estimated to be £80,000.

95 Front page, 3 November, 1951, *Daily Mirror*.

96 Gift of the Gregory family to the Red House archive, Aldeburgh.

97 *The Rape of Lucretia* is now, along with *Peter Grimes*, held in the Red House archive (gifted by Gill, Robert & Elizabeth Gregory) and *Albert Herring* is in the possession of Gill Gregory.

sky studies – at the first Aldeburgh Festival of music in 1948[98]. Carlos Peacock, an art historian and friend of Britten, wrote in his Note to the Exhibition, of Constable having 'the farmer's eye' which could, at a glance, recognise 'all the signs and portents of the land.'

It is perhaps significant that Dr Gregory, the owner of this fine collection of Constable pictures, is himself a farmer whose work in connection with the breeding of Ayrshire cattle has won him international fame.[99]

In 1949, the year of Alexis's bankruptcy, a selection of Constable's sketches and drawings was exhibited at the Arts Council, with an Introduction to the catalogue by the well-known art historian, Sir Kenneth Clark, who comments on the oil sketches being rendered with 'the freshness and sparkle of nature.'[100] The small, sturdy figure of Alexis might be compared with that of a child – a 'fresh'-faced boy, his eyes lit up in excitement, a boy who had left behind a site of terrible trauma and, in his hurry to get on, embraced life and all it had to of-fer, never appearing to look back.

In a letter to Britten from Carlos Peacock, in 1962, he refers to 'the little sea-piece Dr Gregory gave you', which would appear in Peacock's book, *John Consta-ble: the Man and his Work*[101]. This small painting can be seen today on the walls at the Red House in Aldeburgh, where Britten and his lover, Peter Pears, lived. The largest painting in my grandparents' collection was Constable's 'Marine Parade and Old Chain Pier, Brighton', and in 1951, on the cusp of his arrest in Lyons, Alexis's debt was partly relieved by the Treasury stepping in with a £7500 grant to cover half the cost of the painting at £15000, having agreed this with the Tate Gallery trustees, who had purchased the painting in 1950.[102]

The subject of 'the little seapiece' (undated), in Britten's collection, is a tem-pestuous storm at sea, which might be viewed as the modest counterpart of the 'six-footer' the Tate had salvaged. Over half of the very small oil paint-ing is filled with thunderous looking clouds that seem to have just rolled into view. There are hints of blue and the light from the sun is attempting to break through. At the centre of the painting there are two boats and some sea birds

---

98 Sandhills & Prior's Hill (Aldeburgh): John Constable, R.A. (1776-1837), An Exhibition of Oil Paintings, Water Colours and Drawings from the Collection of Doctor H.A.C. Gregory, M.C., Red House archive, Aldeburgh.

99 *The Aldeburgh Festival of Music and the Arts,* Programme Book, Ed Eric Crozier, June 5th – June 13th, 1948.

100 Sir Kenneth Clark, Introduction, 'Sketches & Drawings by John Constable from the Collection of Dr H.A.C. Gregory, MC, The Arts Council of Great Britain, 1949'.

101 1965.

102 26. Jan 1951, 'Treasury Helps to Pay Debts of Wanted Man', *Warwick Daily News*.

being blown by a strong wind. It is a picture of danger, exuberance and resilience. The storm may blow over at any moment.[103]

The picture might be a motif for my grandfather's life at this time – the storm of bankruptcy breaking in 1949 followed by several months in Brixton prison between 1951 and 1952 and then his final release, after which he set up a smaller medical practice in London and prospered.

Hazel moved to *Makepeace Mansions* in Highgate and Basil, a newly qualified doctor, had to find work and build a career quickly. My father's references from the R.A.F., after his posting at the medical unit in Suez, were glowing and ensured his rapid progress as a psychiatrist, becoming a consultant and later Superintendent of Horton Hospital, a large psychiatric hospital in Surrey. In 1962 he was appointed as the first director of the Paddington Day Hospital (NHS) in west London, under the aegis of St Mary's Hospital.

The Day Hospital was a pioneering experiment in group psychoanalytic therapy, following the work of Dr Wilfred Bion and others with traumatised solders during the Second World War. The NHS was founded on the 5th July 1948 and I think my father, who died over forty years later in 1990, would have been greatly saddened by its struggle to survive today.

Hazel lived just three and a half years after the founding of the NHS. She and many other paediatricians had been laying the foundations of the service in their work at the new Infant Welfare centres and in the new paediatric wards in hospitals. Her early death in 1952 meant she did not live to enjoy her retirement – although I suspect she would have continued working for as long as she was able. She had made her mark, though, as a pioneering woman of ambition and high achievement, in a medical world that had fiercely resisted the advent of women doctors.

Her book, *Infant Welfare*, bears witness to her work and that of many others – the doctors, nurses, health visitors and voluntary workers who dedicated themselves to the care of infants and children and their mothers.

*

INFANT WELFARE FOR THE STUDENT & PRACTITIONER BY HAZEL H. CHODAK GREGORY (1926)[104]

In this closing section of the Introduction I shall refer to my grandmother as 'Dr Chodak Gregory' or 'Chodak Gregory'.

Infant Welfare, published in 1926, appeared at a time when, in earlier decades, The Boer War (1889-1902) and the First World War (1914 – 1918) had

---

103 The Red House collection of paintings, Aldeburgh.
104 Hazel H Chodak Gregory, *Infant Welfare for the Student & Practitioner*, London: Lewis, 1926.

highlighted the very poor health of the recruits enlisting. Many steps had already begun to be taken to improve the health of infants and children, leading to the establishment of milk depots and infant welfare centres. The latter gave advice on feeding, general management and hygiene and they also aimed to develop an awareness of the many conditions, which might affect an infant's health, along with the preventive measures that could be taken.

In 1884 the London Society for the Prevention of Cruelty to Children was founded and in 1889 this became the National Society for the Prevention of Cruelty to Children (NSPCC)[105]. In 1889 Parliament passed The Children Act, whereby legal measures were established to protect children from abuse and neglect, with criminal penalties. Even though the Infant Welfare centres were not directly concerned with issues of cruelty and neglect, their development took place in the context of children's welfare being taken much more seriously at this period. Midwives' acts were passed in 1902 and 1905, whereby midwives should have training. Lay women could not stand in their place unless they were supervised by a certified midwife or physician. In 1911 maternity benefits were provided and in 1918 the National Council for the Unmarried Mother & her Child was established. Just two years before *Infant Welfare* was published The Society for the Promotion of Birth Control Clinics had been founded in 1924 to improve the access of working-class women to birth control.[106]

In writing *Infant Welfare* Chodak-Gregory was formalizing and importantly recording the work of the centres at this time of urgent change in improving the lives of children. In 1918 women over 30 had been granted the vote for the first time and throughout the country newly enfranchised women were calling for more infant welfare centres to be established. In 1919 Norwich, where I live, had ten infant welfare centres, providing ante-natal checks and advice, along with distributing milk from dairies and milk with vitamins for babies. They also monitored children up to five. In the journal, *Public Health*[107], the reviewer welcomes Dr Chodak-Gregory's book as 'filling an ancient and desolate gap in the literature',

The position of the Infant Centre doctor is in many ways peculiar to itself, and text books on pediatrics and the ordinary run of hospital experience are far from being a complete equipment for Infant Centre work, and may,

---

105 The Liverpool Society for the Prevention of Cruelty to Children was the first Society founded in 1883.

106 Sadie McMullon, 'A Welfare Pioneer', 107/March 2022, *Social History, Discover Your Ancestors*.

107 *Public Health* is a journal published by The Royal Society for Public Health (RSPH), established in 1856. It is an independent charity dedicated to improving & protecting health in the UK and worldwide. *Public Health* has been published continuously since 1888.

indeed, if unaccompanied by a wide appreciation of all the factors pertaining to child welfare, be of little use in helping the Medical Officer to develop the Infant Centre to its fullest usefulness.

Dr Gregory describes with humorous and sympathetic appreciation the position and the problems of the doctor within the Centre, and emphasizes [...] the importance of his inter-relationship with the other workers, particularly the inter-relationship of doctor and health visitor, which may make or mar the quality of the work that is performed.[108]

There are some criticisms of the book, such as its not developing the discussion of coeliac disease and concluding with a chapter on Infant Mortality. The latter, the reviewer suggests, should have appeared at the beginning of the book. I shall discuss this point when considering the final chapter, 'Infant Mortality'.

The reviewer's description of *Infant Welfare* 'filling an ancient and desolate gap in the literature' resonates. He is perhaps suggesting that the care women have given infants and children down the centuries, along with the knowledge and experience they have acquired, has invariably gone unrecognised as such knowledge and experience have often been passed on orally, from woman to woman and mother to mother, without a written record to 'prove' that their care has been informed and often intuitive, with the added important benefit of such knowledge being acquired through experience.

The first paragraph of the *British Medical Journal* review of *Infant Welfare* begins,

Since Dr Budin[109] established in Paris in 1892, the first infant welfare centre, there has been so rapid a multiplication of such places in this country [UK] that it is almost certain every medical practitioner must have come into contact with them either directly or indirectly.

Dr Chodak Gregory's book, he writes, sets out to inform those who do not have this knowledge and 'to assist those who are embarking upon this work for the first time.' The reviewer welcomes 'Dr Gregory's championship of [the] wisely restricted use of the 'comforter' – 'Doctors who have an intimate personal knowledge of infants and have given thoughtful observation to this much abused object, will doubtless support the author.' As David Stevens has stated, Dr Chodak Gregory was alone among her peers in continuing in post after marriage and having a child. Basil, her son, was five years old when *Infant Welfare*

---

108 287, Vol 39, 1925 – 1926, *Public Health*.
109 Pierre-Constant Budin (1846 – 1907) was a French obstetrician and one of the founders of modern perinatal medicine.

was published in 1926 so his mother did have 'intimate personal knowledge' of an infant.

The reviewer's closing remarks are critical of too much space in the book being 'devoted to treatment' – the 'real function' of the doctor at the Infant Welfare centre, he states, is 'to prevent illness by education of the mothers, and when any departure from the normal occurs in the infants they should be referred to a pediatrist for treatment.'[110]

Dr Chodak-Gregory does make very clear that, in the event of serious illness, the infant should be referred to the pediatrist immediately. 'It is not [...] thought desirable that medical treatment should be carried out to any extent in the ordinary Welfare Centre' but 'it is not always easy to draw the line between the minor ailment and the illness'.[111] The treatments she advises are in relation to the common conditions affecting infants and the many ways in which mothers can prevent and treat these.

The reviewer's reference to one of a centre's aims being the education of mothers highlights the focus on the mother, as the significant parent, which was typical of the period. Mothers, especially working-class mothers, were invariably held responsible for the poor health of infants and the prevalence of infant mortality.

The contribution Chodak-Gregory makes to the development of the infant welfare centres is significant, especially in her focus on preventive work and the vital importance of fresh air to a child's health. Her emphasis on relationships between doctors and nurses and their patients is also important in that, as a much respected, increasingly eminent female professional, her words carried weight with the male establishment that would elect her a Fellow of the RCP in 1934, eight years after the publication of *Infant Welfare*.

The Introduction[112] stresses that work at the Infant Clinic 'is less cut and dried than curative work, especially among children, and perhaps for that reason is all the more difficult for the inexperienced.'

> The first thing to realise is that the atmosphere of an Infant Welfare Clinic is entirely different from that of the Hospital Out-patient Department and that the work has got to be arranged on different lines.

Chodak-Gregory makes a very clear distinction between the Infant Welfare centre's work and that of the Outpatient clinic. Patients arriving at Outpatients will, she writes, come with a definite complaint and will give an account of their symptoms.

110 Ibid, *Public Health*.
111 5, Ch I, *Infant Welfare*.
112 Ibid, vii – xi, *Infant Welfare*.

By contrast the mother arriving for the first time at an Infant Welfare Centre, the centres being a relatively new feature in her landscape, 'has come with mixed motives'. She was advised to attend, as other women were doing, and would, for example, like to know the baby's weight and might be given free or cheap baby supplies – weighing babies and the provision of supplies, especially to mothers living in poverty, were key features of the Centres.[113] She is not necessarily arriving with 'symptoms' to recount.

> It is for the doctor to open the conversation, and it is his business to establish a friendly relationship with the mother, win her confidence as soon as possible, and satisfy himself that the child's daily routine is as it should be, that the feeding, clothing, habits, etc., are such as are likely to keep it in good health. For the doctor is not there to cure children of disease. He is there to prevent disease [...]

The doctor new to this work, she states, will find the first day at the Infant Welfare Centre especially trying,

> The young medical officer has taken his degree, has probably done two or three years of resident hospital work of all kinds, and may have already treated hundreds of babies with whooping cough, diarrhœa, and broncho-pneumonia [...]

But even though the medical officer is by now very familiar, in his hospital work, with the symptoms of disease 'he will find that personality, manner, and an ability to handle people will be worth just as much to him as a theoretical knowledge of pediatrics.' This kind of work, Chodak Gregory emphasises, 'cannot possibly be done in a hurry' and 'the hustling atmosphere of a Hospital Casualty department' is to be avoided.

Doctors today might bear her words in mind in the current atmosphere of extreme stress prevailing in so many hospital settings and in GP surgeries. General Practitioners are all too often (understandably given the heavy workload) in too much of a hurry when examining the patients who are fortunate enough to be given an in-person appointment. Chodak-Gregory also stresses that the doctor should not see more than a reasonable number of babies per session or he will, by the end of the session, 'have given about as much of his energy and vitality as could be expected of him.' It is better for the mother, she adds, 'to have a good heart-to-heart talk with the doctor once in two weeks, or even in three, than to line up with fifty other mothers and get a bare three-minutes interview.'

---

113 The tv series, *Call The Midwife* (created by Heidi Thomas, 2012 – present) gives some idea of an Infant Welfare Centre and the different rooms at such centres. The weighing of babies and supplies of fruit juice etc. are a regular feature in this series.

She does, though, express the prevailing medical view, at the time, of working-class mothers being generally 'ignorant' about infant welfare. But she is ahead of her time in pointing out that the doctor-nurse relationship must be developed on the basis of mutual respect. She is unafraid of pointing out the institutionalised arrogance, which has been a feature of the medical profession.

> Theoretically the nurse is supposed to fall in with the doctor's ideas and see that his advice is carried out, but it would be absurd to expect an experienced woman to have no opinions of her own, and it must be excessively annoying to her, and very trying to her loyalty, to see the young scientist (with little or no practical experience) rushing ahead, not deigning to ask her opinion or discuss a case with her.
> [...] they should together evolve a plan of campaign, allowing them-selves plenty of opportunity for discussion and exchange of views.

Chapters I and II set out the ways in which an Infant Welfare Centre might be set up and managed. The work was still in its early stages with such centres being established increasing rapidly since the early twentieth century. They had been managed by voluntary agencies, Borough and Council authorities and were in the process of being connected to a system of Health Visiting.
Chodak- Gregory draws attention to the importance of the Mother and Child Welfare Act of 1918, which was seminal in that its aim was the betterment of mother-hood and the saving of child life. Under the Notification of Births (Extension) Act, 1915, the 1918 Act extended the care to mothers before, during, and after confinement, and also provided for the supervision of children up to school age.

In the Hansard record of the statements made in the House of Lords on the second reading of the Bill in July, 1918, Viscount Peel emphasises that, with the expansion of measures to improve healthcare for mothers, infants and children, such powers must still 'be exercised through the local authorities.' In setting up committees to institute and implement such powers it was vital, he states, that 'at least two women must be appointed on every maternity and child welfare committee.' He also pays tribute 'to the very admirable schemes' already under foot in places such as Lewisham in London, Huddersfield and Liverpool. His speech concludes,

> [...] if the schemes are carried fully into effect, I believe a great deal will be done in the future to diminish the death rate among children and to repair the terrible ravages which have been made in our population by the war.[114]

---

114 18 July 1918, 981-988, Vol 30, *Hansard* (1803 – 2005), 'Maternity & Child Welfare Bill'.

In his speech the Marquess of Crewe notes 'that with reduction in the rate of infant mortality comes a reduction in the rate of invalidity, and a great deal of suffering, waste, and loss is saved in the future life of those who are thus protected.'[115]

Chodak-Gregory sets out the role of Local Authorities and Voluntary Centres along with details of the Treasury grants to the Centres. She provides an account of the type of building that had been used for the Centres – often houses or shops adapted to the Centre's needs – along with an outline of the required accommodation. The ideal, though, of 'beautifully planned' buildings, 'fitted with every convenience' invariably fell far short in that there was not the money for building schemes, she states.

Throughout *Infant Welfare* 'the open-air life' is promoted and in Ch I, in her discussion of the Health Visitor, Chodak-Gregory recommends the work, which is 'arduous and not too well paid, but interesting' and having the advantage of an 'open-air', healthy occupation, which involves 'a sense of freedom' uncommon to nurses. Every Centre, she writes, should have its own apparatus for 'ultra-violet ray therapy', so long as such 'preventive' treatment does not encroach upon the work of the general practitioner or hospital.

Making the distinction between the role of the GP surgery and the hospitals, and the role of Infant Welfare centres, Chodak-Gregory is careful not to tread on anyone's toes. She was on the cusp of being appointed Physician of the Children's wards at the Royal Free and she is, in a sense, still quietly nodding to the authority of the predominantly male world of medicine.

In each Infant Welfare Centre, Chodak-Gregory states, 'the Medical Officer may be […] a general practitioner, or any qualified man or woman with experience in pediatrics.' She adds,

> A married medical woman is generally well received, as mothers have infinite confidence in a doctor who has borne babies herself. The man and the unmarried woman often make excellent medical officers too, and they have the advantage that they are not constantly tempted to judge other children by their own.

In Chapter II there is a discussion of the 'General Management' of child care outside the Centre. Chodak-Gregory stresses the importance of appointing a visiting nurse, in addition to the health visitor as it was essential that the doctor in the Centre should have a thorough knowledge of living conditions, the size of families, their housing and their incomes. The visiting nurse should aim to

115 Ibid Hansard.

get to know individual mothers and assess their needs. Air and light are emphasized as major health benefits and Chodak-Gregory makes some pertinent points about 'the poorest slum children' having some advantage in that they play in 'the narrow, cobbled streets of East London', by contrast with children in artisan families, with the mother often not allowing her children to play in the street, even when they invariably have no garden or even a backyard. Rickets was still a common disease in the 1920s but a new treatment with ultraviolet lamps – which Chodak-Gregory advises as a necessary feature of infant welfare centres – had been pioneered by the German pediatrician, Kurt Huldschinsky, in 1918-1919, with some successful results.

Rickets is the subject of Ch X, *Infant Welfare*. The condition was beginning to be cured in the 1920s, with the increasing awareness of the role of sunlight and nutrition, especially Vitamin D, in improving infant health. In recent years, though, rickets has reappeared in the UK. In 2019 the number of cases hospitalised was estimated to be the highest for fifty years. There are many factors but a lack of sunlight and poor nutrition continue to be significant factors. Dr Elena Ferguson gave an excellent presentation on 'The History of Rickets and the startling recurrence of the condition' at the Royal College of Paediatrics & Child Health conference in Glasgow, 2025.

Chapter II provides detailed advice on bathing infants, the importance of sleep and clothing. Pain, Chodak-Gregory writes, is often the cause of an infant being unable to sleep. 'The cry of pain sounds very like the cry of hunger and is frequently mistaken for it […]'. Neither must be ignored, she urges. I was a baby and child growing up in the 1950s and my mother adhered to the common practice of ignoring a child's cries unless they were heard during the timetabled feeding time. I was relieved when I first read my grandmother's words.

She does, though, suddenly introduce 'nervousness' to describe a baby's difficulty in sleeping, which does read much less sympathetically. She cites 'heredity' as the main cause of this anxiety, which accords with the late nineteenth, early twentieth-century preoccupation with ideas of a degenerating human race, combined with the rise of eugenics theories. Heredity does play a part but at this period such a diagnosis was aligned with a certain fatalism.

The highly strung child with an ill-balanced nervous system is recognisable from early days […] it is never still, is easily excited, and though tired is often quite unable to get to sleep. Sleep when it comes is apt to be light and easily disturbed. These babies require to live a humdrum life with undeviating routine in quiet surroundings, and to be brought up by placid people.

In Virginia Woolf's novel, *Mrs Dalloway* (1925), Septimus Warren Smith, who has been traumatised by his military service in the First World War, is prescribed a 'rest cure', which Woolf herself experienced at several points in her life when she was struggling with acute mental health issues. Rest cures, at their most extreme, involved nigh total isolation and the patient not being allowed any mental stimulation. Combined with a diet of fatty foods the rest cure often resulted in unhealthy weight gain and depression.[116] In 1941 Virginia Woolf committed suicide as her mental illness was debilitating her yet again. One of the reasons given for her decision was that she could not bear the prospect of going on another rest cure.

Chodak-Gregory's recommendation, for the 'nervous' infant, of 'undeviating routine in quiet surroundings', sounds alarmingly close to an idea of the rest cure and is a jarring note in a book that is largely sympathetic to and in tune with infant needs and with the mother's state of mind. In 1926 psychoanalysis and psychology were still in their infancies but by 1943 Chodak-Gregory was attending a Child Psychology committee at the British Paediatrics Association headquarters in London. The psychoanalyst, Donald Winnicott, was also a member of the committee, which was discussing topics such as psychological problems in childhood.[117]

Hector Charles Cameron (1878 – 1958), a paediatrician and head of the children's department at Guy's Hospital in London, writes in his book, *The Nervous Child* (1919)[118], of the effect emotions and environmental stimuli can have on a child's behaviour and health. He describes 'the teeming activities of the quick, restless little brain' of a 'nervous' child, which can be overlooked by the physician, who may not appreciate the child's state of mind.

In the chapters on 'Breast-Feeding', 'Artificial Feeding' and 'Feeding after Early Infancy (Chs III – V) there is a wealth of detail. Chodak-Gregory presents a balanced discussion of the pros and cons of the different methods of feeding. Ch III begins,

> There can be no doubt that what Nature has provided for the infant is the food that it is most likely to digest and assimilate […] even the makers of artificial foods have the grace nowadays to begin their advertisements by the admonition, 'Mothers, nurse your babies!'

Such an imperative admonition to parents these days would be out of the question, but it is very much the tone of the period. 'If women are to be believed,

---

116 Charlotte Perkins Gilman (1860 – 1935) wrote a short story, 'The Yellow Wallpaper' (1892), based on her own harrowing experience of a rest cure prescribed by Dr Silas W. Mitchell (1829 – 1914), who pioneered the rest cure, primarily for women.

117 Dr Chodak Gregory and Dr Winnicott both resigned from the committee in 1945. I have not been able to discover the reasons for their resignations.

118 H.C. Cameron, *The Nervous Child*, 1919/1930.

there are still far too many general practitioners who advise weaning on the slightest provocation, not realising that a baby who is not doing well on its mother's milk will, nine cases out of ten, do even worse on any artificial food.' Chodak-Gregory is careful to balance this statement with an acknowledgement that some babies thrive on artificial feeding. She does, on the whole, 'believe' the 'women' who report that GPs are too quick to advise early weaning. She strongly recommends 'the open air' as a vital component of the nursing mother's routine. I recently met a young woman, who was born in a chlorine and chemical-free birthing pool out of doors in France[119], where she floated a while before the umbilical cord was cut. My grandmother would, I think, have been impressed.

In Chapter III she comments on the mother's *'State of Mind'* having 'an extraordinary influence on suckling'. She describes 'the ideal mother' as 'the placid, contented woman who refuses to let herself be worried by any untoward event, who moves and thinks with calm deliberation [...] The ideal cannot often be realised.' The word 'placid', though, can often have a negative connotation today, suggesting dullness, monotony and even indifference, but in the 1920s that connotation was not so common. Chodak-Gregory also describes breast-feeding as pleasurable, especially the 'draught' sensation, when the breasts are filling up. The onus, though, is placed on the mother, who was so often taken to task at this time, for not being the ideal. The mother bears the burden of responsibility for whatever might go wrong but, given the pervasive ideology, Chodak Gregory's tone is mostly sympathetic.

In the section on 'Weaning' she describes the nine months taken as a general rule for weaning in the UK, but emphasizes that this period can vary, especially in the case of mothers living in poverty, who were attending the Infant Welfare Centres. The mother's milk, she states, is providing better nutrition than the 'cheap brand of sweetened condensed milk' which the baby will be fed as an alternative. Interestingly Chodak-Gregory regrets the decline of wet-nurses, who were too expensive for Infant Welfare Centres and had lapsed in general anyway, citing the 'hundreds of pints of good human milk running to waste daily' in the event of early weaning.

Chs IV & V continue with very detailed information about artificial feeding and feeding after early infancy. Chodak-Gregory is careful to emphasise how different each individual baby and child can be when it comes to food – with different constitutions and inclinations. She continues to make the point, with some urgency, that 'the hungry cry of a baby is very similar to the pain cry.'

---

119 South Pacific islanders often give birth in shallow sea water. In the UK birthing pools, partly owing to our weather, are less common but many women bathe in warm water during labour for pain relief.

Stools – normal and abnormal – and the dangers of diarrhœa, one of the significant causes of infant mortality at this period, are the subject of Chs VI & VII. Chodak Gregory goes into minute detail in describing the many different kinds of stool and the ways in which foods affect the digestive system of the baby. Several remedies are suggested and the importance of good hygiene is stressed. The same attention to detail is to be seen in Ch VIII on vomiting. Paediatricians today will find much that is still relevant, when world markets are flooded with cheap processed foods and sugar-dense confectionery. As ever it is often those living in poverty who cannot afford to buy the more nutritious foods that constitute a healthy diet.

The opening sentence of Ch IX, 'Premature Infants', startled this writer. 'Prematurity, which is largely responsible for a high infant mortality, is chiefly due to maternal causes.' I first read this as indicative of the extent to which working-class mothers were being blamed at this period for being inadequate. Chodak-Gregory then lists some of the causes of prematurity – trauma, physical or mental, prolonged malnutrition, diseases such as tuberculosis, nephritis, syphilis, diabetes and operations for other than pelvic conditions. The malposition of the fœtus in utero may also be a cause of premature labour.

Chodak-Gregory is not actually saying the mother is to *blame* so much as helpfully identifying the maternal causes. A report on infant mortality and the state of child health in the UK today (RCPCH[120]) states, 'Social inequalities continue to have a marked impact on infant mortality. The risk of infant death increases with greater levels of maternal deprivation [...] Infant mortality trends also show widening health inequalities. The report states that 'government efforts to reduce child poverty remain crucial to improving infant survival.' It also calls for 'improved pre-conception care, including maternal health and education.'[121]

The role of the paediatrician today extends beyond the strictly clinical and pioneers such as Chodak-Gregory were leading the way, a century ago, in their work with mothers, who were invariably doing the best they possibly could whilst struggling with high levels of poverty and deprivation.

In Ch X, 'Rickets', Chodak-Gregory states that there was still much to be learned about the aetiology of the disease. She describes the increasing amount of research being undertaken and provides much detail in listing and describing causes and possible causes, along with remedies to strengthen bones. Chs XI and XII, dealing with 'Rashes in Infancy' and 'Pyrexia in Children', follow and *Infant Welfare* concludes with a chapter (XIII) on 'Infant Mortality'. When I arrived at this chapter, as a non-medical person I found that, after learning about

120 Royal College of Paediatrics & Child Health.
121 RCPCH website.

the many conditions that affect infants, this conclusion took a step back to set out, with statistics and graphs, the key concern of the medical practitioner, at this period, with lowering the rates of infant mortality. Although the reviewer of *Public Health* is of the view that the chapter would be better placed at the beginning of the book, the conclusion actually provides an endpoint at which the practitioner's attention is reminded of the topic that was very much in the public eye at the time and makes sense of the book as a whole.

The clinician today, in her close focus on the infant conditions and diseases presented to her at the GP surgery or walk-in centre, will be reminded of her wider responsibility in maintaining the health of the country's population. Chodak-Gregory records the rates of infant mortality and the declining numbers in her day.

> The rate of Infant Mortality in this country [...] the total rate, the comparative rates in different areas, the causes of death, etc., may be found in detail in the Annual Report of the Registrar General. [...] The infant mortality rate is the number of infants dying under one year of age, per 1,000 of infants born.
>
> The first point to notice is the steady decrease of mortality from all causes during the last thirty years or more. During the years 1891-1900 the annual rates were between 150 and 160; they dropped steadily until in 1913 the rate was 108 per 1,000.

She states that this decline 'has been most noticeable since the Notification of Births Act' in 1907, marking 'the beginning of organised Infant Welfare Work in this country.' Any doubts, she writes, about the enthusiasm of 'the mothers of the country' and 'whether the average working-woman would ever attend the centres for advice about her children', have been set to rest. 'They attend in their thousands, and their willingness to learn is a revelation.' Chodak-Gregory's tone here is a reminder of the rigidity of the class structure at this period. All lower- and working-class mothers are assumed to be ignorant.

By 1923 the rate had dropped to 69 per thousand. In 2024 world rates have been estimated at between 100 deaths per 1,000 to as low as 1.5 per 1,000, drawing attention to just how privileged we still are in this country, the UK rate being estimated at 3.8 per thousand. That said, there are regional differences in the UK and the rates vary, often considerably, in terms of deprivation and ethnicity. As the gap between rich and poor currently widens, infant mortality rates grow higher in deprived areas.

Chodak-Gregory notes that the highest rate in 1923 was in the Northern County Boroughs, 90 for the year, 'while the lowest is 48 in the South Urban Districts'. A graph illustrates five categories, giving the most common causes of death, which include common infectious diseases, TB, diarrhœal diseases, developmental diseases and 'the rest'. There must, though, be an allowance, she writes, for 'a good deal of inaccuracy in the certification in the cause of disease' unless a post-mortem has been performed.

This chapter in conclusion is well-placed in that it draws attention to the urgency of lowering the infant mortality rate further. The country was struggling economically and in the same year, 1926, the General Strike took place in the UK and 1929 would see the Wall Street crash in the US. In the field of infant welfare there was much work yet to be done. *Infant Welfare* is indeed a book that 'fills an ancient and desolate gap in the literature'.

My grandmother would have been somewhat surprised, I think, by the resourcefulness and resilience of mothers living in very cramped and unpropitious circumstances to this day. Mothers – with extraordinary courage and fortitude – continue to struggle with securing the safety and welfare of their children the world over.

*

THE MIND OF THE GROWING CHILD

The Mind of the Growing Child (1928) is a collection of a series of lectures, ed-
ited by Eva Violet Mond Erleigh (1895 – 1973)[122], a philanthropist and children's welfare advocate, who became the President of the National Council of
Women in 1955. The collection includes a lecture by Chodak- Gregory, titled
'The limelight and assertive child' and other essays by educationists, medical
journalists, physicians, psychiatrists, psychologists, psychoanalysts and writers,
many of whom had served with the army during the First World War, gaining
first-hand experience of soldiers suffering from shellshock (war trauma), along
with physical wounds.

There are lectures on a wide range of topics, including daydreams, the effect
of sunlight on a child's psyche, family discipline, fear, heredity & environment,
jealousy, the psychology of infancy and temperament. In 'The Only Child' Donald Winnicott, the psychoanalyst, writes that 'play' with other children will be
key to the only child's development.

The Mind of the Growing Child was also published in New York and, in a review
that appeared in *The Elementary School Journal* (US) in 1929, the writer recommends the collection as benefiting from being written by physicians on topics
that are psychological, whilst bearing in mind 'the physical nature and welfare of
the child'. The book might be read by parents – 'it is in simple and readable language' and it 'may be considered as a work of popular psychology', whilst being
free from 'the usual psychological terminology.' The volume's accessibility to the
lay reader does not preclude it from possessing 'scientific accuracy.'

Psychiatry, psychology and general medicine have developed considerably
since the 1920s but the reviewer's discussion of the importance of assessing the
child's physical condition, in assessing a child's psychological state, cannot be
overstated. Six weeks, say, of Cognitive Behavioural Therapy today (which can
be very effective when the focus is on correcting a specific behaviour or in pain

---

122 Eva Violet Mond Erleigh (Ed), *The Mind of the Growing Child: a series of lectures*, The Scientific
Press, Faber & Gwyer, London, 1928.

management) is still no substitute for longer term, in depth, treatment for more complex mental health conditions.

In the May edition (1929) of the *Wanganui Chronicle* (New Zealand) Chodak-Gregory's lecture, 'The Limelight & Assertive Child', was published.[123] The lecture had been given as one of a series arranged by the National Society of Day Nurseries[124] in London. Chodak-Gregory also lectured on Maternity & Child Welfare between 1928 and 1931 at the Royal Holloway College, which was opened in 1886 by Queen Victoria as an all women college, which became part of the University of London in 1900.[125]

In 'The Limelight & Assertive Child' Chodak Gregory states that 'all children are not assertive' but that every child 'likes to be in the limelight on some occasions.' The child who is 'shy and retiring' in the presence of friends and relations, 'may be found strutting about the kitchen 'showing off' before the cook.' Here she has the middle-class family in mind. Chodak-Gregory argues that love of 'limelight' can become a habit to discourage. She also discusses, with subtlety, the increasing attention being paid to the child at this time,

> For the limelight is but the eye of the observing adult, which is focussed so much more intently on the child now than it was 50 years ago. In most civilized countries and in all classes there has been a general awakening of interest in child-life […] the development of the child mind is watched, its innocent sayings are carefully analysed, its motives inquired into.[126]

Children, she states, now 'join in the conversation as a matter of course, ask for explanations of what they do not understand, and are not shy in giving their opinion on any matter.' Parents study 'the minds of their offspring' and this development can encourage 'the limelight child', aware that he is the centre of the parents' gaze, to rely on too much habitual attention.

---

123 'The Limelight & Assertive Child', Our Babies, p. 10, 109, 9 May 1929, *Wanganui Chronicle*.
124 The National Society of Day Nurseries was a charitable & voluntary organisation set up in 1906 for pre-school aged children in the UK. They also provided specialist two-year diploma qualifications for nursery nurses & childcare nannies and instruction classes for mothers caring for babies and infants.
125 The Royal Holloway College admitted male postgraduates in 1945 and male undergraduates in 1965.
126 Carolyn Steedman discusses the ways in which children became the concentrated focus of the adult gaze in nineteenth-century history & literature. She raises questions about this focus often being more about the adult psyche than that of the child being scrutinized. My review of her book, *Strange Dislocations. Childhood & the Idea of Human Interiority 1780 – 1930*, 1995, appears in 2, Vol 8, *Women: a cultural review* (1997), OUP.

Chodak-Gregory sees this as inevitable and argues that 'at least [he] is not storing up hidden complexes' in that the modern child can be frank, keeping nothing back in the fear of ridicule or blame. She is careful to state that 'his manoeuvres' (conscious or unconscious) are compatible with a 'genuine artlessness and innocence'. Boys and only children are, she states, more prone to seeking 'the limelight'. Her evolving ideas are evident a few years after this lecture was given, in a Presidential Address she gave to the Medical Society on May 18th, 1931[127], on behalf of the London (RFH) School of Medicine for Women, where she would be appointed Vice-Dean a year later. The Address was titled *Physiognomy of Disease in Childhood* and it begins with a discussion of 'visual observation'.

Although the vulgar use of the word Physiognomy is generally applied to the face only, the original meaning includes the art of judging by bodily form as well as facial features, and may be taken in this instance to mean the art of cultivating visual observation in our clinical examination of patients.

[...] If inspection is useful in examination of the adult patient whose facial expression may be masked [...] how much more useful and reliable is the study of childish expression which is rarely anything but genuine and sincere. In infants especially, facial appearances may have to replace history, for whereas in children of five years and upwards there are always two histories to take into account, that of the parent and that of the child himself, in the case of infants only one history is available.[128]

Chodak-Gregory, as in her ideas of 'the limelight child', is keen to emphasise the sincerity of a child's expression. She may have talked with or read papers by the psychoanalyst, Melanie Klein (1882-1960), who was just four years older than her. Klein's *The Psychology of Children* was published in 1932. The 1920s and 1930s was a period in which there was a rapid development of psychoanalytic ideas, in the wake of the First World War, when psychoanalytic work with traumatised soldiers was being pioneered. Klein presented several papers in the Bloomsbury home of Virginia Woolf's brother, Adrian Stephen, who qualified as a psychoanalyst in the late 1920s. Chodak-Gregory, living in Bloomsbury, may well have been present to hear Klein's papers. This was a time when ideas of a child's

127 H.H.C.G., 'Physiognomy of Disease in Childhood', Presidential Address delivered to the Medical Society by Dr Chodak Gregory on May 18th, 1931, *Magazine of the London (Royal Free Hospital) School of Medicine for Women*. No. 109, Vol XXVI, July 1931.

128 Ibid, 'Physiognomy of Disease'.

psyche were the focus of much discussion and Chodak-Gregory is clearly aware of the dangers inherent in too much adult analysis of the child's mind.

Klein's close observation of infants importantly revealed that the baby's development can be seriously affected, even permanently damaged, by her relation to the mother and the mother's capacity for loving engagement. She established a key tenet in psychoanalytic thought that a baby's psyche, in its attempt to comprehend the world, is in a state of splitting in its identification with good and bad objects, the mother being the primary object. If the growing child is unable to overcome the splitting, in the recognition that life cannot be spent veering between 'good' and 'bad' relations to the mother, and is unable to mature, the adult psyche, and its capacity for paranoia and psychosis, will develop abnormally.

I was a patient in Kleinian psychoanalytic therapy for several years and her words often rang true but our contemporary focus on 'authenticity' in human development finds an echo in my grandmother's discussion of an infant's 'expression' being 'rarely anything but genuine and sincere.' The psychoanalytic project has been key to finding my own ways in the world, but it can be too driven by theory and its potential rigidities, which sometimes burden, even entrap the mind of the patient and of the therapist herself. The so-called 'sophistication'[129] of adults, and also of psychoanalysts, can at times undermine, interfere with a child's – and later the adult's – spontaneity and the freedom to express herself. Facial appearances in the infant substituting for 'history', in my grandmother's words, may free the child's mind, and the adult's, from a weight of psychoanalytic interpretation, as well as from parental knowingness, which will have its own biases and preoccupations, often obscuring the experience of the child herself.

*

---

129 A 'sophist' can describe 'a person who uses clever but fallacious arguments', but today the word 'sophisticated' implies an ironic appreciation of complexities – ironic in a post-modern sense that 'truth' is only ever relative.

A NOTE

As the many obituaries mentioned, my grandmother was reserved but quietly and effectively authoritative in her bearing and in her humanity. I am reminded of the dignity with which she bore her husband's fall from grace. When he went so spectacularly bankrupt and was very much in the public eye, his story being followed in the newspapers by the public at large, the shock of discovering, at the age of sixty-three, that Alexis had supported a second family in the wings for ten years or more, must have been devastating. Her death at the young age of sixty-five, two and a half years later, was surely hastened by shock and immense hurt.

In ending her days, living in genteel poverty at Makepeace Mansions in Highgate, I like to think Hazel had chosen this home as a sign of making her peace after the unkindness of events. In her last years, for some months before she died on the 12th January 1952, she stayed with my late parents (who married in July 1949) in Theydon Bois, Essex – in a small, sweet cottage near an avenue of trees.

What a long way she had travelled – from Bloomsbury, and the cultural hub of the 1920s zeitgeist, to Portland Place and flying high in aeroplanes alongside the late and great actor, Ralph Richardson, to *Houghton Grange*, where Hazel and Alexis dreamt of opening a health centre exclusively for people living in poverty and free of charge.

For much of their married life they had been generous, hard-working and at times glamorous partners in their many highly successful endeavours. In writing this Introduction to my grandmother's book I have made new discoveries and many new friends along the way. I am delighted and proud to be related to a pioneer who made her mark on generations to come.

*

INFANT .WELFARE

INFANT WELFARE

FOR THE STUDENT AND PRACTITIONER

BY

HAZEL H. CHODAK GREGORY
M.D., M.R.C.P.

ASSISTANT PHYSICIAN IN CHARGE OF INFANT DEPARTMENT
ROYAL FREE HOSPITAL
PHYSICIAN, EAST LONDON HOSPITAL FOR CHILDREN, SHADWELL

LONDON
H. K. LEWIS & CO. LTD.
1926

CONTENTS

CHAPTER VII

CHAPTER VIII

CHAPTER IX

CHAPTER X

CHAPTER XI

CHAPTER XII

CHAPTER XIII

INTRODUCTION

THESE preliminary remarks are addressed to the medical man or woman who is embarking on work at an Infant Clinic for the first time.

Preventive work is less cut-and-dried than curative work, especially among children, and perhaps for that reason is all the more difficult for the inexperienced.

The first thing to realise is that the atmosphere of an Infant Welfare Clinic is entirely different from that of the Hospital Out-patient Department, and that the work has got to be arranged on different lines.

In the Out-patient room the patients have come for some definite complaint, and the formula " What's the matter, ma'am ? " or " What are you complaining of ? " will let loose a flood of symptoms and complaints which have been prepared and discussed with neighbours in the waiting-hall. Very different is the case at the Welfare Centre, where the child's mother has come from mixed motives— she was advised to, other women did, she wanted to know the baby's weight, she thought she might get something cheap. She has nothing definite to complain of, and she says nothing as she seats herself by the table with her plump baby on her lap. It is for the doctor to open the conversation, and it is his business to establish a friendly relationship with the mother, win her confidence as soon as possible, and satisfy himself that the child's daily routine is as it should be, that the feeding, clothing, habits, etc., are such as are likely to keep it in good health. For the doctor is not there to cure children of disease. He is there to prevent disease, and in order to do so he must be on such terms with the mother that he may control and direct, as far as circumstances permit, the upbringing of the child.

There are probably few experiences so trying as that first day at the Infant Welfare Centre. The young medical officer has taken his degree, has probably done two or three years of resident hospital work of all kinds, and may have already treated hundreds of babies with whooping cough, diarrhœa, and broncho-pneumonia. But this is a fresh experience, and he will find that personality, manner, and an ability to handle people will be worth just as much to him as a theoretical knowledge of pediatrics.

It must be fairly obvious, though unfortunately it is not generally recognised, that this kind of work cannot possibly be done in a hurry. No good work can be accomplished in a Welfare Centre which has the hustling atmosphere of a Hospital Casualty department, nor can we expect a woman, who has never been taught to express herself lucidly and concisely, to confide the details of her infant management and ask those questions to which she really does want an answer, when she is aware of a crowd of mothers sitting impatiently outside and longing to get home.

The young mother with her first baby, ignorant though she may be, is often the most inarticulate.

She knows practically nothing about babies, except a few amazing facts told her by her grandmother, and in most cases she is willing to learn and very trustful ; but it takes some little time to plumb the depths of her ignorance, as she is often blissfully unconscious of there being anything wrong at all. With such we cannot be too thorough, nor be afraid of instructing her in the very simplest details.

It follows that every medical officer of a clinic should make some definite rule as to how many babies he will see at one session, and having decided on a particular number, he should firmly resist any efforts to make him see more, except in cases of real urgency. A good average number is twenty, and this will probably include five or six quite new cases. By the time that twenty mothers have been interviewed, twenty babies examined, details of feeding discussed, daily habits inquired about, advice given in the most tactful manner possible, and all entered duly upon the records, a period of from two to two and a half hours will have passed, and the doctor in charge will have given about as much of his energy and vitality as could be expected of him.

At flourishing centres with good attendances, there should either be frequent sessions or a large staff of doctors, and if this is impossible for financial reasons, the mothers should content themselves with occasional interviews with the doctor, and depend meanwhile on the advice of the visiting nurse. They will generally admit that it is better to have a good heart-to-heart talk with the doctor once in two weeks, or even in three, than to line up with fifty other mothers and get a bare three-minutes interview.

Another most important point is that the doctor and health visitor should work harmoniously together. There are many ways of conducting these centres and there is room for a great divergence of opinion in the matter of infant feeding; the only possible way to run the clinic successfully is for doctor and nurse to have one main policy, and stick to it.

Theoretically the nurse is supposed to fall in with the doctor's ideas and see that his advice is carried out, but it would be absurd to expect an experienced woman to have no opinion of her own, and it must be excessively annoying to her, and very trying to her loyalty, to see the young scientist (with little or no practical experience) rushing ahead, not deigning to ask her opinion or discuss a case with her. Rather, the scientific knowledge of the doctor should be combined with the practical experience of the visiting nurse, and they should together evolve a plan of campaign, allowing themselves plenty of opportunity for discussion and exchange of views.

It is important for anyone who is to deal with children in health and disease to get a clear idea of normal conditions before proceeding to study the abnormal; unfortunately, however, such simple and obvious matters as the examination of human milk, macroscopic and microscopic studies of infants' faeces, an examination of healthy infants' bones as they appear in a radiograph, are not generally included in the medical student's curriculum. The Infant Welfare doctor must acquaint himself as speedily as possible with these fundamentals, if his work is going to be useful, and although he will probably have neither the time nor the opportunity to analyse milk, he at least will know the appearance of it, and will be able to reassure the young mother who, on seeing it for the first time, is afraid that the thin bluish stuff " cannot be doing her baby any good " ; and though he may not be able to pursue the chemical investigation of an infant's fæces, at least knows the amount, colour, consistency, etc., to be expected at various ages. Indeed the stool gives such an excellent indication of what the gastro-intestinal tract is doing—and that tract is so much the most important organ at an early age —that one can hardly consider an infant truly and thoroughly examined without an inspection of the latest soiled napkin.

INFANT WELFARE.

CHAPTER I

THE MANAGEMENT OF A WELFARE CENTRE

MANY Welfare Centres have grown up within the last twenty years, some managed by voluntary agencies, others by Borough and Council authorities. At first unconnected, at least officially, with Health Visiting under the Notification of Births Acts, they have now been made part and parcel of the system of Infant Welfare Work all over the country.

THE MOTHER AND CHILD WELFARE ACT, 1918

This Act drew together the tangled threads of voluntary and rate-aided work for mothers and infants, and gave wide powers to local authorities to evolve varied schemes for the betterment of motherhood and the saving of child life. At the same time practical help in the shape of Treasury Grants was promised towards schemes approved by the Local Government Board, which was at that time at the head of affairs of health.

Whereas previous work, under the Notification of Births (Extension) Act, 1915, had concentrated on the welfare of infants for a few months only, the

I

1918 Act extended the care to mothers before, during, and after confinement, and also provided for the supervision of children up to school age.

COUNCIL CENTRES

At present the majority of Welfare Centres are under Local Authorities, and are managed by a Mother and Child Welfare Committee. This committee was made a statutory one by the Act, that is to say any Council undertaking welfare work was obliged to have such a committee; its members were to be partly composed of Council members, but one-third must be drawn from outside, and at least two members must be women. Though the work is generally undertaken by County and Borough Councils, there is nothing to prevent the District Councils from having their own schemes, but these should not interfere with the larger schemes; they are as a rule not advisable, as being uneconomical.

VOLUNTARY CENTRES

Many of the old voluntary centres, pioneers of the system, are still run with great success, especially in London. These are generally managed by Committees of ladies who give their services and make themselves responsible for collecting funds. New centres may be formed, but it is of course desirable that they should not interfere with, or overlap, the work of the Local Authorities. Accordingly it has been laid down that such centres can only be recognised and subsidised by the Ministry of Health if there seems to be a real need for them in the districts concerned, if they will co-ordinate with the work of the Local Authorities, and will be prepared to keep satisfactory records. Recognised voluntary centres must be open to inspection by Officers from the Ministry of Health. These conditions apply to Centres attached to Voluntary Hospitals, often run in connection with the hospital maternity department ; they are especially valuable at Teaching Hospitals, as the study of Infant Welfare forms an indispensable part of the curriculum of a medical student.

GRANTS

Treasury grants to all approved centres are at present at the rate of 50 per cent. on total expenditure. The grant paid in each year is assessed on the basis of expenditure incurred in the preceding financial year.

THE CENTRE

One would like to be able to build new Welfare Centres for children. They could be beautifully planned and fitted with every convenience. There is, however, not enough money for building schemes at the present time. The organisers of a centre have to be content with adapting a house or shop for the purpose. The expense of adaptation and equipment of such a place may be partly met by a grant from the Treasury if the plans, estimates, etc., have been previously approved by the Ministry of Health.

The minimum accommodation required is : (1) a large waiting-room ; (2) a smaller room, well-warmed, for undressing and weighing babies ; (3) a doctor's room ; (4) lavatory accommodation. There must be also a shed outside for prams. This much is essential. There may also profitably be :

(1) a room where older children may play while waiting for their mothers; (2) a room divided into cubicles for suspected cases of illness: mothers ought not to attend Welfare Centres with children suffering from rashes, sore throats, etc., but they do, and will probably continue to do so: any suspicious case should be isolated from the rest until the doctor has seen it—such cases should be seen and disposed of early; (3) a room for ultra-violet ray treatment; (4) a massage room; (5) a dispensary.

DENTAL CLINICS

It is an immense advantage to have a Dental Clinic in connection with the centre, preferably established in the same or an adjacent building. This should be available both for mothers and children, and is especially useful in Pre-natal work, as attention to the teeth is an important part of the hygiene of pregnancy.

THE OBJECTS OF A WELFARE CENTRE

These may briefly be stated to be :
1. The maintenance of a good standard of health in the infants and young children of the district.
2. Education of the mothers.
3. Treatment of minor ailments.
4. The early detection of disease.
This work is carried out partly by the full-time work of the health visitor, partly by the Doctor's Clinics held regularly at the Centre, and partly by the institution of classes and lectures for mothers.

The workers should keep before them the primary aims of their undertaking, and should never allow the centres to degenerate into depots for the distribution of infant foods at wholesale prices, and, difficult though it may be at times, they should try to keep the centres free from association with the giving of material relief.

CASES OF ILLNESS

In the following pages indications for the treatment of various unhealthy conditions will be found, as many of the subjects would have been incomplete without such a reference. It is not, however, thought desirable that medical treatment should be carried out to any extent in the ordinary Welfare Centre ; once babies are definitely ill, it is better from every point of view that they should be treated by the general practitioner or the hospital physician. It is not always easy to draw the line between the minor ailment and the illness, and the Medical Officer is naturally tempted to deal with cases of illness in his own Welfare babies when he knows himself quite capable of doing so ; but directly ill children are encouraged to attend these centres, they become a danger to the healthy babies, and immediately the primary object of the Welfare Work is destroyed.

THE MEDICAL OFFICER

The Medical Officer of the Infant Welfare Centre may be an Assistant M.O.H., a general practitioner, or any qualified man or woman with experience in pediatrics. A married medical woman is generally well received, as mothers have infinite confidence in a doctor who has borne babies herself. The man and the unmarried woman often make excellent medical officers too, and they have the advantage that they are not being constantly tempted to judge other children by their own.

Whoever he is, the doctor must attend regularly. The plan of having a rota of general practitioners of the district to serve each for a few weeks at a time, in order to hurt nobody's feelings, is, of course, ridiculous.

THE HEALTH VISITOR

This individual is appointed by the Local Authorities in the case of a Council Centre, by the Managing Committee in the case of a Voluntary Centre. In either case she is responsible to the M.O.H. for the district as well as to the doctor for whom she works.

There is no standard examination for health visitors. Certain alternative qualifications, which are not compulsory, are laid down as desirable, and at the present time most visitors hold at least two of these. They are :

1. A General Nursing Training.
2. The certificate of the Central Midwives Board.
3. A Sanitary Health Certificate.
4. A certificate of an approved society for Training Health Visitors.

Only exceptionally is health visiting done by qualified medical women.

The work is arduous and not too well paid, but it is interesting. The open-air life is healthy and there is a sense of freedom which is not common to all nursing appointments.

The Health Visitor, variously called the " Visiting Sister," the " Lady Superintendent," the " Visiting Nurse," should if possible be allotted a district of such a size that the average number of births per annum does not exceed 250–300. This may seem a small number, but in view of the fact that she must visit from time to time till each child is five years old, it will hardly be possible for her to deal with any more.

Her function begins when that of the midwife ends. As a general rule she visits midwives' cases as soon after the tenth day as possible, doctors' cases after the fourteenth day.

She must be present at every clinic, and should preferably be in the room while the doctor interviews the mothers, for unless she hears the advice given she will find it difficult to work hand-in-hand with him. Often, before an interview, she will be able to give the doctor useful information about the next mother, the kind of home she lives in, the food she really does give the baby, and so on. Her presence adds immensely to the value of the doctor's work, but of course she can only manage this if she has good helpers outside who are capable of weighing babies correctly, giving out the record cards, and keeping the mother happy.

Most of her time is spent in visiting. As her numbers steadily increase she will find it impossible to visit every family regularly, but will make a special point of seeing new babies, first babies, prematures, cases where the mother's milk is threatening to fail, artificially-fed babies, ailing babies, and all those specially consigned to her care by the doctor-in-charge.

If she has the right personality for her work, she will soon be known and sought by all the mothers of her district. They will often come to her for advice which they hardly care or dare to ask of the doctor ; she should, therefore, have an " at home " hour every day, a time when they know she can be found in her office, ready to listen or to talk, to treat a minor ailment as the case may be.

Voluntary Workers

There is plenty of work for the unpaid worker even in the Borough and County Centres. The rates and Treasury grant supply salaries for the doctor and health visitor, and occasionally for other officers, but in a busy centre there remains much work which cannot be paid for, and for which one is thankful to have voluntary helpers. A regular worker can give out record cards, weigh babies, play with toddlers, and talk to mothers.

The *educational side* of the centre too may usefully be organised and carried out by them. Classes in needlework and plain cooking, lectures on hygiene, etc., are much appreciated by the mothers and as a rule well attended. The doctor and health visitor have little time for these, but one or other of them should give a general superintendence to the educational side, in order to see that garments are made to correct patterns, and sound advice is being given on subjects of health. Lectures must be given in the simplest language, not made too dictatorial, and should be flavoured with sound common sense and a recognition of practical difficulties.

Artificial Sunlight

Every clinic should have its own apparatus for the administration of ultra-violet ray therapy. Neither the installation nor the upkeep is very expensive, and the working of the lamps is extremely simple.

The treatment does not encroach upon the work of the general practitioner or hospital, as it is essentially preventive. Heliotherapy is yet in its infancy, but already it has shown remarkable results in cases of rickets, marasmus, tuberculosis, etc., and may be used with great benefit for all ailing babies, especially those whose circumstances and surroundings make it impossible for them to get their share of ordinary sunlight.

Supply of Milk and other Food to Nursing Mothers

There is generally some local scheme in every borough for the supply of milk or dinners to necessitous mothers, either free or at a low price. The food is supplied on the certificate of the Medical Officer of the centre which the mother attends. Milk may also be supplied to children under eighteen months old, or to older children who are in special need of it, e.g. in cases of rickets. This expense falls chiefly on the rates and the Treasury.

Observation Cots

In some places one or two small wards are established in connection with the Welfare Centre, where babies may be admitted for observation when it seems desirable to have their feeding under direct supervision for a little while. Cases of actual illness should not be admitted. It is undoubtedly useful to have these cots, but unless an adequate nursing staff can be supplied, it is better not attempted.

CHAPTER II

GENERAL MANAGEMENT

PERHAPS the most difficult part of the duty of the Clinic Medical Officer is the giving of advice about the general management of the child, apart from the actual feeding.

It is essential that he should first have a thorough knowledge of the living conditions of the people he has to deal with, the size of their families, their housing accommodation, their incomes. Here, the visiting nurse will help him ; she knows which are the poor homes, which the dirty homes (not by any means always the same) ; she soon gets to know the individual mothers, and can tell which are the ones who may be relied upon to carry out orders. With this knowledge gained, the doctor may more easily enter into the mind of the clinic mother, and will be able to give her advice that it is possible to follow. Nor must he be too diffident in offering advice upon general matters, because it is upon the details of upbringing that a child's welfare may depend.

AIR AND LIGHT

The problem of giving children enough fresh air and sunlight is often more difficult than that of providing them with food. The parents at least understand that a child must be fed, but they often think it is a little fussy, if not dangerous, to make such a point of open air. In this matter, the poorest slum children often have the advantage; from the time they can toddle they are turned out into the streets, and play happily in the gutter all day long. The narrow, cobbled streets of East London are full of them. But go one step higher in the social scale and you find the respectable, hard-working artisan's wife, who will not let her children play in the street, has no garden, perhaps not even a yard to her own house, and has little opportunity for spending several hours a day in taking them out herself. There are many women who never go out except for the brief half-hour's daily shopping, and their children stay indoors with them until old enough to go to school.

This problem is a difficult one to solve, but the mothers are generally willing to do their best once they are made to realise the important part that light and air play in the maintenance of health. Many cases of rickets are seen at Infant Welfare Centres in babies who are not suffering from a diet deficiency, but who are living constantly in a dark and stuffy atmosphere.

As for ventilation of homes, anyone who has had any practical experience of the homes of the poor realises how bad that is. At least every mother now knows the right answer to " Do you keep your windows open ? "; and although her reply is not always strictly truthful, it is a step in the right direction that she knows what is correct and healthy.

BATHING

There is a certain amount of prejudice against bathing babies twice a day; it is, nevertheless, a cleanly habit and cannot do any harm. It should be encouraged wherever there is time and means. The habit of oiling new-born babies instead of bathing them in water has been adopted by some obstetricians with a view to lessening the risk of chill. The practice may be usefully followed in the case of premature infants with low vitality, but it is unwise to deprive the normal infant of the hot water, which is cleansing and stimulating at the same time. The risk of chill is a real one when the nursing is careless, but it may be reduced to a minimum if the preliminary washing is done rapidly and the child dried and dressed in a warm room free from draughts. The temperature of the bath should be about 100° Fahr., but clinic mothers do not possess bath thermometers and usually test their water with the sensitive skin of the elbow. The majority tend to give it too hot. A good plan, in the case of inexperienced mothers, is to let the visiting nurse take round a bath thermometer and let them " get the feel " of the water which has been brought to the correct temperature.

Soap should be of the mildest variety and need not be used at all on the face. Powder may be used to complete the drying, but not as an excuse for insufficient use of the towel. It should be a plain starch powder, dusted on finely and immediately stroked off again with the dry hand. One frequently finds babies with masses of sodden powder in the groins, the skin shining red and sore. The buttocks should not be washed after every motion, merely cleaned and dried, the exception being in cases when irritating acid stools are being passed.

As soon as the child's skin is strong enough to

stand rubbing with the towel, instead of dabbing, the use of powder may be discontinued.

There should be as little interference as possible with the eyes, nose, ears, and mouth when a child is being bathed. The custom of poking pledgets of cotton wool or a twisted handkerchief into the nostrils and of wiping out the mouth with the finger, is a bad one, and may do much harm. The *Mouth* will keep itself clean, and is not likely to get infected so long as the nipple and bottle teats are clean and the baby is not allowed to suck its own or someone else's dirty finger. *Thrush* is the most common infection during the first few months, a rapid growth of colonies of *Oidium albicans* over tongue and buccal mucous membrane. The parasite is also able to grow in the bowel, and frequently does so, causing diarrhœa with irritating stools. The favourite home remedy is glycerine of borax, but this is not so quickly efficacious as a fairly strong solution of bicarbonate of soda rubbed gently over tongue, gums, and inner surface of cheek; the parasite cannot grow in an alkaline medium.

As soon as the teeth appear they should be cleaned regularly, especially the double teeth, which are deeply pitted and offer safe lodgment for particles of food. It would be well to keep a stock of small tooth-brushes at Welfare Centres to sell to the mothers in the hope that some small proportion of them might be used for the purpose for which they were intended.

The *Nose* is a delicate organ and should be left alone as long as the child is well, only visible particles of dirt or dried mucus being removed. When catarrh occurs it is chiefly in the naso-pharynx, which cannot in any case be reached, so no attempt should be made to swab out the discharge. Nasal breathing is, in infants, an instinct which it takes months or years of chronic adenoids to eradicate ; even when they breathe through the mouth during waking hours they tend to return to nasal breathing directly they are deeply asleep. When catarrh is present, blocking of the air-way may be very distressing, and it is permissible to induce sneezing by placing a few grains of powdered soap (such as Hudson's) just inside the nostril. As soon as the child is old enough to understand, it should be taught how to blow the nose properly.

Sleep

The healthy, well-cared-for infant, having regular feeds and plenty of fresh air, spends the greater part of its time asleep, often remaining quite undisturbed by surrounding noise.

Many factors may interfere with normal sleep. The chief of these is discomfort from gastro-intestinal disturbances. Flatulent distension and colic are almost invariable accompaniments of dyspepsia in infancy, and these symptoms either make the child's sleep disturbed and uneasy, or prevent it altogether. The cry of pain sounds very like the cry of hunger and is frequently mistaken for it, with the result that many a dyspeptic infant has its condition rendered far worse by the administration of frequent extra feeds. Hunger must not be ignored as a possible cause of sleeplessness, however, and it may be found either that the breast-milk is failing, or, where artificial feeding is being employed, that the mother is ignorant of the appropriate amounts to use. Other kinds of pain are rare in extreme infancy (except the occasional accidents of wounding by unguarded pins), but when teething begins there may be considerable wakefulness, the gums being swollen and sore, and if one can judge from the sudden starts and cries, pain occurs from time to time in sharp stabs. Later, otitis media may be a hidden cause of pain, or there may be the well-known " starting pains," due to relaxation of an early tuberculous joint. Later still rheumatic arthritis may cause pain at night.

" Nervousness," though a vague term, must be used to describe the cause of sleeplessness in a large number of babies. This is not generally a direct fault of environment ; rather heredity seems to be to blame. The highly strung child with an ill-balanced nervous system is recognisable from early days, and it suffers always from a want of repose. It is never still, is easily excited, and though tired is often quite unable to get to sleep. Sleep when it comes is apt to be light and easily disturbed. These babies require to live a humdrum life with undeviating routine in quiet surroundings, and to be brought up by placid people.

In connection with sleeplessness mention ought to be made of that bugbear of all Infant Welfare workers—the *Comforter*. This much-abused but useful article requires a champion. It is true that fat, placid babies, who wake but to feed and sleep again, have no need of such an artificial aid to slumber, and it would be the greatest pity to force it upon those who do not want it. Just as wrong is it to thrust it into the mouth of a crying babe without taking any trouble to ascertain the cause of the cry. But there is no doubt that the comforter is a most useful means of taking the difficult baby over the border-line of sleep.

The nervous baby mentioned above, who is easily tired but cannot lose consciousness, gets more and more weary and fretful every minute that sleep is postponed. Let him have a few comforting sucks, and the border-line is crossed; as sleep deepens, the comforter falls out of his mouth or may be taken out. He will, of course, form the habit of sucking a comforter at his sleep times, and indeed should be allowed to associate it only with sleep; but the habit is easy enough to break at the end of the first, or during the early part of the second, year, far easier than the habit of thumb-sucking or blanket-sucking, which so often takes its place. The comforter may be thrown away when the mother thinks fit; the thumb never can. It seems to be an ineradicable instinct of infants to suck, and it is certainly a soothing process. If they must suck something, let it be a clean rubber comforter that can be boiled daily and washed frequently. The fingers are often dirty and cannot be boiled; they become sodden and sore from the process of sucking, and the habit remains into later childhood. The blanket or nightdress is worse, as a considerable amount of wool is swallowed. Theories about the production of adenoids, the alteration of the shape of the jaw, or the ruin of the teeth are theories only, and remain entirely unsubstantiated.

Facts must be faced. Mothers are certainly going to use comforters for their babies so long as the whole family sleeps together in one room. Would it not be wiser to teach them to keep the comforter clean, boil it daily, refrain from moistening it in their own mouths or dipping it into the condensed milk, and train the baby to associate it with sleep ?

CLOTHES

In a book written for the medical profession it is unnecessary to go into great detail on the subject of children's garments. One assumes that the Infant Welfare doctor has a general idea of hygienic clothing. He must not himself, however, assume such knowledge on the part of the mother, and, although in many centres the infants are brought in already undressed to see the doctor, he should make a habit of asking to inspect clothes from time to time, especially when there is any tendency to chest trouble, sweat rashes, etc., and his visiting nurse should keep a careful eye on this side of the work.

A few difficulties may be pointed out and suggestions made. *Long Clothes* are not absolutely necessary, and it would be more economical to put infants into knitted woollen garments for day wear, using a shawl for the outer wrapping. But since long clothes are a precious mark of social status, and since, when properly made, they do no harm, the point need not be pressed.

A rather faddy method of making all the garments to fasten up along the front, so that they may be adjusted without turning the baby over, is not to be encouraged. It is very good for the baby to be

turned over a few times in the course of its toilet—
it is the only exercise it gets.

The wide, stiff, white binder is not yet dead,
in spite of the combined efforts of the medical
and nursing professions. It still turns up from
time to time, strongly recommended by the old
granny, who says it " strengthens the back." There
is not a word of good to be said for it, and it must
go.

The flannel binder, which acts as a bandage,
while the cord still requires a dressing, is generally
kept in use long after the cord is off. It is not a
satisfactory garment ; firstly, because owing to the
shape of the trunk the binder tends to slip up to
the thorax, leaving the abdomen uncovered and
impeding thoracic respiration ; and, secondly, because it is inexpansible (whether sewn, tied, or
pinned), and is, therefore, an unsuitable covering
for a part of the body which must vary considerably
in size, according to the stage of digestion, amount
of intestinal gas, etc. The knitted woollen belt
is infinitely preferable, and any tendency to slip
up towards the chest may be counteracted by
catching the lower border in the napkin pin.

From the time the child is short-coated it is
usually over-clothed. That is to say, its chest is
over-clothed, while the buttocks and thighs are
hardly covered at all. If there is any tendency to
chest trouble, the clothing is increased still more,
and it is a common occurrence to see a child, brought
up with a cough, being gradually peeled of a coat,
dress, cardigan, three petticoats, two vests, and
lastly a thick layer of cotton wool (in permanent
use). The buttocks, meanwhile, may be covered

by a pair of thin cotton drawers, but these have only been put on for the occasion—at home it sits naked on the floor, probably because its habits are still dirty, and it is so much easier to wash a linoleum floor than a pair of drawers. This unhappy combination of a compressed, over-loaded chest and chilly buttocks must be a strong etiological factor in the production of catarrhal diseases in young children.

CHAPTER III

BREAST-FEEDING

THERE can be no doubt that what Nature has provided for the infant is the food that it is most likely to digest and assimilate. About this question there can be very little difference of opinion, and even the makers of artificial foods have the grace nowadays to begin their advertisements by the admonition " Mothers, nurse your babies ! "

Happily, in the poorest classes, breast-feeding is the rule, because it is the cheapest method of feeding, and because it generally staves off a future pregnancy. The baby who suffers most is the child of the fairly well-to-do artisan's wife, who, in her ignorance, takes the first little attack of gripes or flatulence as evidence that her milk is not suiting it, and turns to the artificial food so convincingly advertised in the local trams, which, she feels, must have so much more " body " in it than plain milk. If women are to be believed, there are still far too many general practitioners who advise weaning on the slightest provocation, not realising that a baby who is not doing well on its mother's milk will, in nine cases out of ten, do even worse on any artificial food. One certainly meets every now and then with the baby who upsets all one's notions about what is proper and right by triumphantly flourishing on artificial feeding after going steadily downhill on breast feeds, and this in spite of an abundance of perfectly good breast milk. These are generally the babies of nervous or much worried women, who seem quite unable to settle down into the calm and cow-like placidity which every nursing mother should strive to adopt.

These rare exceptions, however, do not affect the general rule that every attempt should be made to promote breast-feeding, and that in no case should weaning be lightly undertaken in the early months.

CARE OF THE NIPPLES

During pregnancy the nipples must be kept clean, and any tendency to retraction must be counteracted by gentle pulling movements. Between the advice to harden the skin by bathing with alcohol and to soften it by anointing it with oil or ointment, a safe course is to leave it alone. In any case, there will be tenderness during the first weeks of lactation when the little hard gums snap on to the root of the nipple, but this gradually wears off and the skin becomes less sensitive. Cracks and fissures do appear in some patients, but it is doubtful whether any previous treatment could prevent them.

Treatment of such fissures is best carried out by the application of a 5% solution of silver nitrate, or a few drops of Tinct. Benz. Co., followed by a mild ointment, such as Ol. Ric. ʒj, Ung. Acid. Bor. ad. ʒj.

During lactation the nipples should be kept clean and free from dried milk, which forms an excellent pabulum for micro-organisms. They should be gently bathed after every feed with a pledget of wool soaked in glycerine of borax. As, however, the regular cleansing of nipples at each feed is extremely unlikely to be carried out by the majority of mothers attending an Infant Welfare Centre, it is as well to lay stress on what they really can do—viz. the washing of the breasts at least once in the twenty-four hours with soap and warm water.

Diet of the Mother

Much has been written about the diet of the mother during lactation, and various articles of diet are extolled—from the old wife's stout and milk mixture to the modern enthusiast's concentrated foods and potted vitamines.

Common sense and a knowledge of physiology, however, suggest that it is not so much desirable that a nursing mother should have this or that article of diet as that she should have a mixed diet with a good representation of all the natural food elements, and that, above all, it should be food which she is accustomed to and knows that she can digest. Milk is in itself an excellent food as it contains all the essential elements, but it is by no means a necessary article of diet, and women who find it difficult to digest, as many do, should not attempt to take it. Local authorities are beginning to realise this point, and in some boroughs now the Welfare Centre doctor may order, alternatively to free milk, free dinners for the destitute mothers.

Meat or fish or some equivalent protein food is necessary. It is generally found that lack of protein in the mother's diet leads to poverty of fat in the milk.

Fresh fruit and vegetables are much advocated

at present by reason of their being rich in vitamines ;
but there is something to be said for the old-
fashioned idea of taking these particular articles of
diet sparingly, as there are certainly cases in which
green stools and griping pains can be traced to
oranges, apples, carrots, turnip-tops, etc., in the
mother's diet. Highly spiced foods should also
be avoided.

Some women never drink enough, and these
should be reminded that water is quantitatively the
chief constituent of mother's milk, and they should
make a point of drinking a tumblerful between
meals. Alcohol is unnecessary.

Drugs should be avoided as much as possible.
Iron and strychnine do not seem to affect the
milk, and a tonic of this kind is often valuable
in stimulating the appetite ; but aperient drugs
are nearly all upsetting to the baby, the only safe
one being liquid paraffin. Maternal constipation
in the few weeks after confinement being almost
entirely a matter of weak muscles and consequent
rectal stagnation, a daily enema is really better than
the use of aperients, until normal function is
restored.

Exercise in the open air is an important part of
the routine of the nursing mother, but is all too
often neglected by the busy woman, who confines
her open-air activities to a little hasty shopping
every day. Hard muscular work or anything tending
to overtire her will be likely to check the formation
of milk.

The *State of Mind* has an extraordinary influence
on suckling. The ideal mother is the placid,
contented woman who refuses to let herself ibe

worried by any untoward event, who moves and thinks with calm deliberation, and who concentrates herself for the time being on her maternal functions to the exclusion of all other matters. The ideal cannot often be realised.

The worrying mother is never a good nurse, and even when her state of mind does not actually diminish the supply of milk there seems to be some mysterious influence at work which actually impedes the child's progress, a malign influence which cannot be explained by either the quantity or quality of the milk supplied.

QUANTITY OF BREAST FEEDS.

The capacity of an infant's stomach, though very small at birth—about 1 oz.—increases rapidly, and by the end of the first month a thriving infant is capable of taking 3 to 3½ ozs. at a feed. It is not, however, always necessary for it to have as much as that, and the amount will vary with the number of feeds it is taking in the twenty-four hours.

Charts of food amounts given according to a baby's age are misleading, as a child should be fed rather by its weight than by its age. A good, rough calculation of the amount to be taken during the twenty-four hours is a sixth or a seventh of the child's body-weight; the former is a generous amount. This rule holds good between about the third week and the eighth month; before that it will not take as much—afterwards it will not need as much, because it will be starting on farinaceous foods as well. The weight alone, however, is not always a good criterion of the amount of food that can be taken, as the much-wasted child of eight months old will take considerably more than a three-month child of the same weight. This applies more to artificial than breast-feeding, and will be alluded to again in a later chapter.

Intervals Between Feeds

One's grandmother suckled her baby every two hours during the day, and generally slept with the child and gave it *carte blanche* to feed as it liked during the night. Times have changed. A generally accepted feeding interval now is three hours during the day for the first three or four months (according to the size and vigour of the child), then every four hours. One feed during the night is generally required for the first month or two, though there are healthy, thriving babies who will sleep from 10 p.m. to 6 a.m. without a feed, from birth onwards. If the infant will sleep eight hours at night, it may be left to do so, but it is inadvisable to insist on that interval of abstention if it clamours against it.

It will be seen that the infant will start by having seven feeds in the twenty-four hours, and by the time it is four months old these will have been reduced to five. Test feeds taken at this time will reveal that it amply makes up in quantity what it loses in frequency. There are exceptions to these general rules. Some fat and placid babies flourish best on four-hourly feeding from the first ; while at the other end of the scale there are hungry little wasters who seem unable to take much at one time, and must be fed two-hourly. Babies with evidence of pylorospasm (see page 98) must also be fed more frequently, especially as the condition is usually accompanied by hyperchlorhydria. The premature baby has a very small capacity, and nearly always needs two-hour feeding in the early weeks.

Length of Feed

Fifteen to twenty minutes should be the time of the ordinary feed. The greedy little person who fills himself up in ten minutes will have frequent motions not fully digested, and likely to make the buttocks sore; he should be discouraged and made to take at a reasonable pace by withdrawing the nipple at intervals. More trying are the babies who fall asleep after the first few minutes and cannot be aroused to take more. If they persist in this habit they may have to be fed more frequently for a short while. This somnolence is only temporary, and in a week or two they will be more awake and eager to take full feeds.

Regularity of feed times is of great importance, and the sooner the child gets into the fixed daily routine the better; the brain, the stomach, and the bowels are all trained at the same time. It is even advisable to wake a sleeping babe for a feed rather than break the routine, though of course there are exceptions to this rule, as, for example, during an exhausted sleep after a bad night. In actual practice, it is found that a baby who is supposed to be taking feeds at 6, 9, 12, 3, 6, and 9, is really having the first at 5 and the last at 10 or 11; but this does not matter much as long as he makes a habit of it.

Thirst in an infant, apart from hunger, is probably

quite a frequent sensation, especially when the child is kept in a warm, dry atmosphere. It is advisable from the first to give regularly a few ounces of slightly sweetened warm water, once or twice a day. A woman who has been suckling her baby at night and is trying to break him of the habit should be advised to have a bottle of water ready-boiled at bed-time, and kept warmly wrapped up, so that he may at least have an opportunity of quenching his thirst when he wakes up and cries. The water must only just taste sweet; a common fault is to add too much sugar, a possible cause of fermenting, acid stools, with consequent sore buttocks.

FAILURE OF LACTATION

This in the early days is probably much more frequent than it need be. It is very likely to threaten when the mother first gets up and goes about her work, and the greatest care should be taken at this period to keep the breast functions healthy and active. The diet should be carefully supervised, a tonic given if the appetite fails, and a galactagogue, such as the proprietary preparation Lactagol, may be advantageously administered. Gentle massage of the breast stimulates the circulation in the gland, and may indirectly encourage the formation of milk. The mother should be informed that the chief stimulation to milk formation is suckling, and that a half-empty breast is less likely to fill up again than a wholly empty one. It behoves her, therefore, if she finds it necessary to use both breasts at a feed, never to start the child sucking at the second breast until she is quite sure the first is well emptied. In this connection it must be remembered that breast milk is richer in fat as the gland is drained than it was at the beginning of the feed, so that it is doubly important that the last part of the milk flow should be used.

Mothers often talk about the " draught," and to them this sensation is evidence that the breasts are filling up. The " draught " is a pleasant, tingling feeling in the breast, occurring from time to time during the day, probably a vasomotor phenomenon, and possibly connected with a sudden dilatation of the vessels, which may precede activity of the gland.   There is no real evidence, however, that this sensation has any connection with the formation of milk, and it is certain that many nursing mothers never feel it at all.   It is well to know this, as some women get depressed if they feel no draught and immediately assume that their milk is failing.   They may be reassured.

Supplementary Feeds

During the first two or three weeks of suckling, the flow of milk is not always fully established, and the amount available is not quite enough for the child ; the flow also tends to lessen during the first few days that the mother leaves her bed.   Attention should be given to the diet of the mother, and galactagogues used if necessary ; but even when these measures are successful, as they generally are, it may be necessary for a short time to give supplementary feeds to satisfy the baby's wants.   A simple, easily digested food with little residue should be chosen.   As there is no question of weaning the child, and as about three quarters of its food will be mother's milk, a lack of vitamines or an insufficient fat-content in the one or two extra feeds will be of little importance. For this reason a condensed milk is probably the best supplementary feed, and less upsetting than any other. Happily in the vast majority of cases this supplementary feed can be discontinued very soon.

A different problem is the supplementary feeding resorted to in the case of older infants, say, at the fourth or fifth month. These are (a) those in which the mother's milk, though abundant enough in the morning hours, tends to get scanty in the afternoon and evening; and (b) those in which, although there is enough milk, the mother wishes to be released during the afternoon hours for work or social engagements.

In either case full breast-feeding is not likely to be re-established, and as it will be a natural thing for the child when weaned to continue taking the food given as a supplementary, care should be taken that this contains the food elements in proper proportions, and adequate vitamines.

There are some who believe that, even when there are no such reasons as the above for supplementing, one bottle a day should be introduced in the early months in order that the child may get accustomed to foreign milks in case its mother should suddenly get ill and rapid weaning have to be undertaken. This practice is risky, as there are far too many cases of infants who, having been put on to one or two bottles a day, refuse the breast altogether. Indeed, that is the great risk of supplementary feeding; the bottle teat is much easier to suck than the mother's nipple, and although, no doubt, most babies will take both for months, there are quite a number who will turn from the breast once they have experienced the delights of the bottle. To lessen this risk a teat with a small hole should be used.

Supplementary feeding (except in the early weeks or towards weaning time) is, therefore, only advised in cases of necessity.

WEANING

The period of time for which the infant is suckled is found to vary considerably in different countries and different climates. In Japan the babe is still at the breast at the end of the second year, and in our own country breast-feeding was continued for a much longer period in olden days than it is at present. In these days, nine months has been fixed upon as a useful period for suckling, but such a period is of course quite arbitrary, and although it makes a good general rule, it may be varied with circumstances. The first three or four months are the most trying to the infant digestion, and the mother may congratulate herself if she can keep the child entirely free from artificial feeding during that time at least. After that the dangers are not so great, although it is certainly advisable to continue with the breast milk for a longer period if possible.

Breast-feeding should not be continued after the first year, at any rate in this country ; it is not good for either mother or child, and a large number of cases of rickets is found in children who have been suckled too long. The signs of rickets do not generally develop while the child is still at the breast, but usually a few months later, and can, perhaps, be accounted for by the fact that a child fed long on mother's milk does not take readily to cow's milk, and, in all probability, takes nothing but tea and water as beverages when finally weaned.

On the other hand, when working at an Infant Welfare Centre, attended by the very poor, it is well not to be too insistent on punctual weaning. The milk that the mother is providing is, at any rate, better than the cheap brand of sweetened condensed milk which the babe will have to share with the rest of the family if it is weaned.

Women will be inclined to maintain lactation as long as possible in the hopes of preventing another pregnancy. Lactation, of course, does not actually prevent conception, but it makes it less likely to occur ; conception, however, can take place during lactation even when menstruation has not been re-established. It is certainly not necessary to wean by reason of reappearance of the menses, though the infant may be upset for a few days, and it is not even always necessary to wean for a pregnancy, though it is inadvisable to carry on after the first three months.

In no case should weaning be carried out during very hot weather ; generally the weeks between the middle of July and the middle of September are the most dangerous period, as it is then that epidemic diarrhœa is so prevalent.

Because a child is to be kept on breast milk for nine months, it does not follow that that is to be its only food. From about the seventh month, when it should have cut one or two teeth, farinaceous food may be begun in small quantities. Details of this feeding are given in the chapter on artificial feeding.

The actual weaning should be gradual, and may be spread over a month. Bottles gradually replace the breast feeds, and when it is finally decided that no further breast feeds are to be given, the breasts are tightly bound, saline purges given, and the mother, in most cases, must look forward to forty-eight hours of acute discomfort. On no account must she use the breast-pump or attempt to express the milk—it will only prolong the agony. Some babies are fed with a spoon or cup as they refuse the bottle after weaning. This should not happen if the child has been accustomed to the bottle for water feeds from its early days. It is far more difficult to get babes to take adequate amounts of milk from a cup or spoon than from a bottle.

Wet-Nursing

Not much need be said on this subject in a book especially written about work in Infant Welfare Centres, because, unfortunately, the employment of wet-nurses is not a matter of practical politics in these centres, as they are too expensive. It is a great pity that wet-nursing has been allowed to lapse so much in this country ; it is rarely taken advantage of, even by those who can well afford it. There are naturally difficulties and drawbacks, but they can usually be overcome, and are well worth overcoming for the sake of the great advantage to be gained by supplying human milk to infants during the early months of life. Premature infants especially, who for one reason or another are unable to get milk from their own mothers, have their chances of life trebled if they can be nursed by a healthy foster-mother.

Many American Infant Hospitals have registers of wet-nurses who can come and live in for a period, women who can suckle two or even three delicate premature infants, while their own healthy infant lives partly on the bottle and partly on the " strippings " from its mother.

The baby visiting the Infant Welfare Centre can have no such advantages, but it is sometimes possible for a friend or relation who lives near enough to offer at least partial breast-feeding to a delicate infant. A large proportion of mothers produce more milk than their babies really want, and it does seem a pity that in every town there should be hundreds of pints of good human milk running to waste daily, while any number of unfortunate infants are having their digestions burdened by artificial feeding.

BREAST-FEEDING OF PREMATURES

Premature infants are often extremely backward in learning to suck ; they are also sleepy, lethargic, and feeble. In consequence they may often fail to take the required amount of milk during the day, although the supply is plentiful. Frequent test-feeds should be carried out to ascertain how much the infant is actually taking, and every endeavour made to get the feeds up to an adequate amount for its age and weight. A good plan of procedure is the following : Weigh the infant, put it to the breast, and let it take what it will, helped occasionally by gentle stroking movements on the cheek. When it refuses to suck any more, take it off and weigh again ; then empty the breast either by manual expression, or by the breast-pump. If the weighing indicates that the feed has been inadequate, make it up to the proper amount by feeding with the expressed milk, using either a small spoon or, better still, a glass dropper, such as is used to fill a fountain pen, with rubber teat and rubber end.

Even if the child has taken as much as could be expected, judging according to weight, the breast should still be emptied, otherwise there is inadequate stimulation for milk formation, stagnation in the breast, and often a rapid failure of lactation.

If the infant is quite unable to suck, feeding must be entirely carried out by expression and the use of the dropper ; but this method is not often successful for long, as lactation is difficult to keep up when there is no sucking stimulus at all. It is so important, however, that these babies should be fed on human milk, that every effort should be made to keep the breasts active. The best way to accomplish this (though not always practicable) is for another baby to lend its services, as neither pump nor manual expression can compete with a vigorous healthy baby in keeping up a continuous flow of milk in the breasts.

Manual expression of milk has the advantage over evacuation by pump in that it is more natural, and tends to keep the flow up longer. It is, however, more difficult, and is an accomplishment which has to be practised and acquired, like the milking of cows. The fingers are placed on the underside of the breast below the nipple, the thumb above ; the thumb approximates the fingers by a downward and forward movement of gentle pressure to the base of the nipple ; here a rather sudden " nipping " movement is made between thumb and fingers, and the milk spurts out of the orifices ; the nipple itself is not touched. The milk should be collected in a sterile glass receiver ; with a little practice the breast can be emptied completely by this method.

CHAPTER IV

ARTIFICIAL FEEDING

THE study of the artificial feeding of infants is a very fascinating and a very heart-breaking one. Let it be said at the outset—there is no royal road to infant feeding, there is no perfect artificial food yet discovered, and no two babies behave the same with the same treatment. How best to compound a substitute for the infant's natural food has been the study of pediatrists for many years, yet it is doubtful whether we are any nearer the solution of the problem. True, infant mortality is considerably lower than it was twenty or thirty years ago, but this must be ascribed to education, improved cleanliness, and, above all, to the general care of child life which has been such a marked feature of the last two decades.

Progress in the study of artificial feeding has, unfortunately, lagged far behind the general progress of Child Welfare. Although much work has been done on the subject, the results have been most unsatisfactory. Every effort has been made to produce a food as nearly like mother's milk as possible, usually with cow's milk as a basis; but even when the various elements, proteins, carbohydrates, fats, salts, are given in correct proportions, there remains the fact that the constituents of cow's milk were designed for the stomach of the young calf and not for the human baby. So that success depends on whether the baby's stomach can adapt itself to a strange food or not. We still have with us, and perhaps shall always have, the baby that thrives and grows sturdy on a diet which outrages all the principles of dietetics. We also have the marasmic, atrophic infant that seems quite unable to make use of the most carefully planned and well-balanced nourishment that is prepared for it. The latter has two possible ends. It either dies of intercurrent infection, affecting the gastro-intestinal tract, the lungs, the meninges ; or, after several months during which no weight is gained and apparently no progress made, it suddenly starts behaving like other children, gains steadily every week, and by the time it is two years old, may have actually caught up to the normal child in weight and strength. The food that it happens to be taking at the time that the improvement begins is naturally thought by the inexperienced to be responsible for the good result. But when the same food tried on the next marasmic baby fails to produce the same effect, it is realised that in all probability the change had little or nothing to do with the particular kind of nourishment which was being administered.

The same may be said for the pathological investigations of wasting babies. Given a marasmic without diarrhœa and with fairly normal stools, analyses of the excreta and comparisons with the food intake generally show that the capacity for absorption of the various food elements is unimpaired. It would appear, therefore, that this type of child can digest and absorb, but cannot make use of the food thus gained to build up body tissues.

General Principles

With few exceptions artificial feeding is based on the milk of the cow.

Ass's milk is actually nearer to the human variety in point of proportion of the various elements, containing much the same amounts of protein and sugar, but deficient in fat. It is difficult to obtain and need not be considered as a practical question. Goat's milk is more easily obtainable and may safely be substituted for cow's milk if necessary.

It is unfortunate that cow's milk should differ in so many respects from human milk, not only in the proportions of its various constituents, but also in their chemical constitution.

Both kinds of milk vary considerably in different individuals and at different times, but a rough average comparison is as follows :

	Human Milk.	Cow's Milk.
Protein	1·5%	3·5%
Caseinogen	·75%	2·5%
Lactalbumen	·75%	1·0%
Fat	3·5%	3·5%
Carbohydrate	7·0%	4·0%

The preponderance of *caseinogen* in cow's milk is the first difficulty that the artificially fed baby has to cope with. It is at least three times more abundant than in human milk, besides having probably a different bio-chemical composition ; it is clotted by rennet into a solid, cheese-like curd, and must offer considerable difficulties at first to the child's digestive apparatus. Yet it is surprising how soon the average child gets accustomed to this foreign protein, and how quickly the gastro-intestinal tract adapts itself to its digestion.

Protein indigestion is not nearly as common as was formerly supposed. When white curds show in the stools, one must not jump to the conclusion that they are lumps of undigested casein. Much more often they are fat curds, and although these are not always easy to distinguish by the naked eye, the microscope will reveal the difference. *Lactalbumen*, which forms 50% of the total protein in human milk, is the more valuable protein of the two, as it is richer in cystin, leucin, lysin, and tryptophane, and therefore proportion-ately more nutritious for the growing child.

The *Fat* of cow's milk is in much the same propor-tion as that of human milk, though in both the percentage varies greatly with the time of milking, the individual, etc. It is, however, a different fat or combination of fats, containing less olein and more stearin and palmitin. Physically, too, it is different, the fat globule of cow's milk being coarser and about ten times bigger than that of human milk. This makes it difficult for the child to deal with at first, and probably gives trouble more often than the bulky casein curd.

The *Carbohydrates* are present in decidedly smaller proportions than in human milk, and here again, although both the substances are called lactose, there is evidently some chemical difference in their composition.

The *Salts* also differ. Iron and potassium salts are well represented in human milk ; sodium, magnesium, and calcium salts better in cows.

Vitamines. Both the fat-soluble A (anti-rachitic)

vitamine and the water-soluble C (anti-scorbutic) vitamine are present in fresh cow's milk. The former is more stable, the latter fairly easily oxidised, especially if exposed to high or prolonged temperatures in the presence of air. Unfortunately, the presence of these elusive substances cannot be established either qualitatively or quantitatively by ordinary chemical tests; at present the only tests are biological ones which are laborious, costly, and inexact.

Use of Cow's Milk

Feeding on plain cow's milk is the method of choice for all those babies who cannot get mother's milk. Although much may be said against the use of wet milk, it still holds first place when compared with any other artificial food. It certainly does not bear a close resemblance to human milk, but it is a complete food, containing all necessary food elements, a food which in its natural state contains abundance of vitamines, and one to which the majority of babies can readily become accustomed when given in the right way.

The methods of milk collection and distribution in this country leave much to be desired. The only two kinds of milk on the market which are comparatively clean and reliable are those labelled " Certified " and " Grade A." Between these two there is only a slight difference; they are both taken from herds certified to be free from tuberculosis, in both the conditions of milking (including housing and care of cows, special pails, methods of collecting, etc.) have been certified and are liable to frequent inspection. The difference is in the delivery ; " Certified " milk is bottled at the farms and carried in bottles to town, while " Grade A " milk is sent in large sealed cans to town, and bottled at bottling centres which are also inspected and certified.

The difference in cost between the two methods of delivery is considerable and accounts for the difference in price. Unfortunately, both are much more expensive than ordinary milk, which is collected from any cows, milked under a variety of conditions, and sent to town in cans from which it is distributed in open tins. " Grade A " milk varies in price in different localities, and is anything from 2d. to 6d. a quart dearer than the ordinary milk, but this is partly because clean methods in milking are still somewhat experimental and only a comparatively small number of farmers have introduced them. It may not be within the bounds of possibility to get rid of tuberculosis among cows for many years yet ; the difficulties are great in a country where it is impossible to keep cattle out-of-doors in the winter, not from any delicacy on their part, but for fear of cutting up the rain-sodden meadows. But it is quite practicable to establish a really high standard of cleanliness in the stabling and washing of cows, in the personal habits of the milkers, and in all the paraphernalia connected with the production and distribution of the milk, from the time it leaves the cow to the time it reaches the consumer. If all farms could be brought into line, in these respects, with the nucleus of model dairy farms which have been started all over the country, the chief objections to the use of wet milk would cease.

The *Bacterial* contamination of milk is the greatest

drawback to its use for infants. In the first six hours after milking, the bacterial content is comparatively small—say 12,000 to 18,000 per c.cm. in milk collected under good conditions. After this the multiplication is rapid, and within twelve hours there are more than ten times the number if the milk is neither cooled nor treated, but kept at a moderate temperature. An endless variety of bacteria may be found, with varying pathogenicity. Many are quite harmless, such as the *b. subtilis* ; others only harmful when present in large numbers, such as *staphylococci* and some of the *streptococci*. The most important, and most frequent, are *streptococci* of the lacticus group, which are responsible for the souring of milk, and bacilli of the colon type, some of which are proteolytic. The *b. tuberculosis* occurs in about 10% of all ordinary milk specimens. The sporing types of bacteria cannot be destroyed even by temperatures above boiling point, but the non-sporing types are destroyed fairly readily.

Pasteurisation of Milk can be carried out either in the home or on a large scale commercially. The term is somewhat loosely used, and there are wide differences both as to the temperature to which the milk is carried by this process and as to the period for which this temperature is maintained. Generally speaking, the term implies that the milk is heated indirectly by a water-jacket, the water is brought to a temperature between 60° and 70° Cent. and maintained there for twenty minutes at least. The milk probably never rises quite to the same degree reached by the water, but is only a very little below this. Subsequently, the milk is rapidly cooled. The latter process is particularly important in that (*a*) organisms are not all totally destroyed by pasteurisation, and (*b*) any subsequent contamination by bacteria will lead to a very rapid growth in milk treated in this way, unless the temperature is kept low.

The process of pasteurisation is almost imperative for milk which has to be carried a long way and may not reach the consumer for thirty-six or more hours after milking (unless it can travel in refrigerator vans), and as a matter of fact, most of the milk sold in this country as ordinary dairy milk is actually pasteurised in order to prevent it from going sour, but is not necessarily labelled as such. Unhappily, the principles of cleanliness are not in the least understood by many who work the pasteurising plants, and as a result the milk after treatment often contains almost as many bacteria as it did before. Home pasteurising is generally carried out by heating a vessel of water which contains bottles of milk already diluted and modified according to the child's needs. It is difficult to keep the water at an even temperature for twenty minutes without standing by and watching it the whole time. If the process is properly carried out, the bacterial content is considerably diminished (e.g. from 65,000 to 15,000 per c.cm.) Whether the tubercle bacillus can be surely destroyed or not is a matter of doubt. Sporing organisms can certainly not be eliminated, as the spores are resistant to a much higher temperature than that of pasteurisation.

BOILING OF MILK

Much experiment has been carried out on the use of boiled milk for young animals, and many observations made on its use for babies. As a result, there is a general opinion that boiling for short periods, or " bringing to the boil," does not interfere with the nutritive value of the milk and does not destroy the vitamines.

Certain changes occur in its physical qualities; some of the calcium is thrown out of solution—this only brings it on a level with human milk, which contains less calcium; albumen is precipitated—not a disadvantage, as it is probably rendered more digestible thereby; there is some delay in clotting with rennet and a decrease in the viscosity of the fat : altogether it may be said there is a slight increase of digestibility of boiled milk over raw, while the nutritive value remains much the same. It should be added as a practical point, that whereas very young infants will nearly always take boiled milk quite well, older children frequently dislike the taste and refuse to take it.

The advantage of boiling is, of course, the comparative sterilisation which is obtained. Prolonged boiling would make milk safer still from a bacterial point of view, but this must be avoided, chiefly for the sake of the vitamines. Even the short process of " bringing to the boil " is enough to diminish considerably the bacterial content, especially the *streptococci*, certain of the *coli* group and the *tubercle bacilli* ; most of these are destroyed, leaving a variety of non-pathogenic bacteria and some putrefactive organisms.

The terms " Sterilised milk " and " Nursery milk " are both misleading and should be forbidden. " Sterilised " implies a condition impossible for any milk on the market, wet or dried, and as the

word has no official recognition, there is no standard
of cleanliness to which milk labelled in this manner
must be kept by the retailer. " Nursery milk "
is a term which suggests good quality and cleanliness
to the average consumer ; actually, it has no
practical advantage over any other milk. Inquiry
generally elicits the information that " Nursery
milk " is the ordinary milk taken from cows at the
retailers, strained to rid it of gross dirt, and delivered
in bottles. As this entails extra handling, with
the further risk (a very lively one) of contamination
with unclean hands, unclean bottles, etc., the last
stage of the milk is worse than the first. The
writer, in her innocent youth, once suggested
the use of " Nursery milk " to a mother. The
woman smiled a peculiar smile, and said, " Oh no,
Doctor ! You see I've worked at a milk shop."

Administration of Cow's Milk

At whatever age an infant is to be fed with cow's
milk, it is as well to begin with a generous dilution.
It is a mistake to suppose that the degree of dilution
must vary with the age of the child ; it must rather
vary with the time which the child has had to adapt
itself to the digestion of a strange milk. Once the
digestive mechanism has been adapted to cope with
the proteins, fats, carbohydrates, and salts found in
cow's milk, the need for dilution ceases, although
many infants never get on to completely undiluted
milk, but do better with a slight admixture of
water, say 1 in 5 or 6 of milk. The chief reason
for the preliminary dilution is to lessen the amount
of thick casein clot that forms in the child's stomach
when the rennin begins to act. There may be

considerable difficulty at first in the digestion of
these curds, which may give rise to vomiting or to
curd diarrhœa. A dilution of *1 part of milk to
2 parts of water* brings the total content of protein
rather below that of human milk, and the amount
of caseinogen to about the same. This is a good
proportion to begin with, and as tolerance is
gradually established, equal parts of milk and water
may be used, then more milk than water, and so on,
until whole milk or nearly whole milk is being used ;
the rate of progress varies with individual infants
and does not depend on their age ; careful examination of the stools gives the best indication for
increasing or decreasing the proportion of milk.

Then the addition of sugar must be considered.
Cow's milk has a smaller content of sugar than
human milk, so that even when given whole, a
slight addition is necessary. When diluted, there
will be a considerable shortage of sugar. Taking
7% as the normal standard of carbohydrate in
human milk, and 4% as that of cow's milk, it is not
difficult to calculate the amount of sugar to be
added to any given dilution of cow's milk. Lactose,
or milk sugar, is, theoretically, the correct kind of
sugar to add, as it is approximately the same substance as the lactose of human milk. There is not
much advantage to be gained by using this instead
of cane sugar ; commercial lactose is rather expensive, and not very sweet ; both lactose and cane
sugar are disaccharides, and have to go through
much the same process of fermentation, though
with different ferments ; their nutritive value is
probably the same. The addition of sugar is
generally carried out in a most haphazard manner,

some mothers being in the habit of adding a tea-spoonful of sugar to any sized feed of any dilution ; excess of cane sugar is a common fault and sometimes leads to fermentative diarrhœa. In the feeding of marasmic infants, the percentage of carbohydrate may sometimes be increased with advantage, but in that case dextrin or maltose or both are added rather than cane sugar or lactose.

ADDITION OF FAT

If the food requirements of infants are to be gauged by the proportion of elements in the mother's milk, then diluted cow's milk will require an addition of fat. But here we have to go very carefully. That part of the cow's milk which an infant tolerates with the greatest difficulty is the coarsely globuled fat which is so different, chemically and physically, from that of its mother's milk. Its first experience of cow's milk will generally result in the passage of fatty lumps in the stools (often mistaken for protein curds), even when the milk is diluted and no extra fat added.

If the correct percentage be made up by the addition of cream, the result may be rapidly disas-trous. It is a good practice, when prescribing milk feeds for an infant who has hitherto had no experience of raw milk, to start with a low percentage of fat in the milk, and, watching the stools carefully, take them as an indication for gradually increasing the amount. Healthy babies are extraordinarily adaptable, and the passage from diluted to whole, or nearly whole, cow's milk need only take a few weeks. On the other hand, some babies never tolerate cow's fat very well, and it may be advisable

in order to give a sufficient amount of fat to add to
the food other forms of fat which can more easily
be digested. Cod-liver oil is one of the most
useful, especially as it is known to be rich in fat-
soluble vitamine. It may be made up in a 50%
emulsion, and either added to the bottle, or if it
seems to make the food unpalatable (and even the
youngest infant has its own opinion about the taste
of its bottle), it may be given separately.

Various fatty compounds such as Vitoleum
Cream, Virol, Roboleine, etc., have been introduced
of late years for use in the feeding of infants : some
are fat emulsions, others are combinations of fats
and malt. Animal and vegetable fats are frequently
combined, the animal variety being chiefly from
butter, eggs, and marrow; the vegetable from nuts.
The manufacturers generally aim at producing an
easily emulsified fat, with melting power as near
to that of human milk as possible. They have a
very useful place in infant and child feeding, as it is
not always easy to find fats which are well borne, and
cod-liver oil, though most valuable, is not tolerated
by every child, and is not by itself a real substitute
for the fat of human milk. They are, however,
dangerous food-stuffs in the hands of an ignorant
public, as many of them are widely advertised and
are used indiscriminately for all kinds of marasmus,
irrespective of the fact that many of the wasting
conditions of infancy have their origin in fatty
diarrhœa.

It is a common practice to add citrate of sodium
to the milk, gr. iij to gr. vj, in a feed, as this salt
renders the curd more soft and flocculent ; but it is
quite unnecessary to continue this practice in-

definitely; after a few weeks the citrate may be safely omitted, as by that time the child's internal economy has learnt to deal with the cow's caseinogen.

Peptonisation is another method of overcoming the curd difficulty, and, although not very fashionable at present, it is really extremely useful in the early stages of weaning. A peptonising powder containing pancreatin is added to the milk at blood heat and allowed to act for from ten to twenty minutes; the milk is then brought to the boil rapidly, to prevent further action. It is slightly bitter even when peptonised only for a short time, but most babies will take it when sweetened, and it is generally effectual in putting an end to curd indigestion.

Malted Wheats, or "Infant Foods," may be considered here, as they are not, and are not supposed to be, complete foods for babies, but are used in conjunction with cow's milk. They are all cereal foods, some completely malted, i.e. with their starches changed to dextrine and maltose, others incompletely malted, with a certain proportion of unchanged starch. The former include such well-known foods as Mellin's, Mead's Dextrimaltose; the latter include Benger's, Savory and Moore's.

Again, malted wheats are often combined with dried milks; of this variety of food Allenbury's 1 and 2, Hooker's Malted Milk, Mead's Re-co-lac, are examples. This last class is, of course, made up with water, not with milk. Finally, there are foods composed of completely unaltered starch; these are not fit for infant consumption, but there are, unfortunately, plenty in the market.

4

The completely malted wheats have a definite value in feeding the youngest infants. Dextrin and maltose are readily converted in the infant's intestine, and while possessing the same nutritive power as sugar, have a higher energy and heat-producing value. Such a "food" may, therefore, be used to replace or partly replace sugar, the amount used being the standard 7% of carbohydrate, or, in some cases, rather more. The presence of dextrin and maltose in milk has the advantage of rendering the protein clot more flocculent and so more digestible.

The partly malted wheats should not be used for the youngest infants, as it is a good rule not to use unconverted starch before, at any rate, the fourth month (most observers say the sixth). Benger's food is an exception to this rule, as it contains pancreatic ferments, proteolytic and diastasic, which act during the process of "bengerising," so that the milk by the time it is ready has little if any free starch in it and makes a soft flocculent curd in the stomach. This preparation, indeed, makes an extremely good stepping-stone to the use of raw milk for babies who are first rather intolerant of the curd. Theoretically, it would be the same to peptonise the milk and add a little dextrin and malt, but this method is easier and makes a more palatable drink than peptonised milk.

It is not necessary to continue this food for long ; the period of "bengerising" the milk may be gradually reduced from twenty minutes to five, and by the end of a month the child will, in most cases, tolerate milk quite well. Not that there is much harm in continuing the administration of these preparations, always provided that the resulting mixture does not contain too high a carbohydrate content. The harm done in the use of malted wheats has generally arisen from the careless, haphazard way in which they have been given. The ignorant mother so often has the idea that milk is too " thin," and what the baby wants is a " good, thick, nourishing food." Consequently she mixes in the carbohydrate till it has the consistency of porridge, quite regardless of the instructions on the tin; and not recognising that milk is the important item of the food, has probably already diluted that freely. It is not surprising that children fed in this way get rickets.

The foods consisting of entirely unconverted starch are still all too prevalent; they are responsible for much infantile dyspepsia, diarrhœa, and rickets.

Barley water, frequently used as a diluent instead of plain water, contains about 1% of starch, and is comparatively harmless. It is sometimes useful as it modifies the curd in the same way as dextrin and maltose, producing thereby a finer curd, and also acts as a mild purgative, but it cannot be said to be nourishing, and as poor mothers nearly always make it badly its use is not recommended as a routine.

Unfortunately, nearly all so-called infant " foods " are advertised in such a way as to give the impression that the milk with which they are made up is a comparatively unimportant part of the feed, the truth being, of course, that milk provides the main part of the nourishment, the " food " being an addition which may or may not be useful. It will be seen therefore that, while prescribed with care and exactitude by the medical and nursing professions these preparations may be useful adjuncts, especially with delicate infants, they may prove a real danger to the ignorant and credulous.

Dried Milks

Since its introduction, some twenty years ago, the manufacture of dried milk has increased enormously, and there is now a very large variety of preparations in this country, and indeed all over the world. Many of these are genuine attempts at the production of a clean, digestible food made from the best milk, and in some cases adapted or " humanised " to meet the infant's needs before the process of drying. Others are absolute frauds, being prepared from skimmed milk or from stale leavings of the dairy no longer fit to be sold raw.

There are two quite different processes of preparation, the Roller method and the Spray method.

By the *Roller method*, the milk is drawn in a fine layer over rollers or drums filled with super-heated steam ; the milk is dried instantaneously, after reaching a temperature of about 206° Fahr., which is maintained for only a little over three seconds ; by that time the roller has brought the dried film of milk to the opposite side, when it is scraped off by a knife edge lying across the drum ; the film falls into a covered collector. The method has the advantage of sterilising the milk to the point of killing tubercle bacilli, lactic acid bacilli, and most of the pathogenic organisms. Sporing bacteria remain, including some non-pathogenic forms, such as subtilis, and some pathogenic forms chiefly of the colon group. The bacterial count from milk of this variety, taken as it comes off the roller, is an exceedingly low one ; the subsequent bacterial count (from the dried product when tinned) depends entirely upon the methods of handling after the drying process. Manufacturers who use the roller process claim that as the film of milk is covered by a layer of steam during the few seconds exposure to a high temperature there is no oxidisation, and therefore no destruction of vitamines. These two points, viz., the comparative sterility and the retention of vitamines, are very important. The drawbacks to this method are, that the dried powder is not very easily soluble and the reconstituted milk gives a poorly emulsified fat, which tends to rise to the top in large, yellow globules.

By the *Spray method*, the milk is atomised in a fine spray in a chamber of heated air. The temperature never exceeds about 160° Fahr. The resulting product is a readily soluble powder, with unchanged lactalbumen and easily emulsified fat. Its physical properties have the advantage over dried milk of the roller process. On the other hand, there are disadvantages.

It is not so free from bacteria as the roller-dried milk (many brands contain about 10,000 per c.cm.) ; it will not keep so long, but becomes rancid, partly owing, perhaps, to its increased exposure to air during the drying process and to the inclusion of a core of air in many of the dried particles ; finally, it is questionable whether the anti-scorbutic vitamine remains intact. Manufacturers suggest that there is an advantage in having a large number of lactic acid organisms retained in dried milk, as they will by their growth, when the milk is reconstituted, tend to keep down the numbers of proteolytic organisms which cannot grow in an acid medium. The chief drawback to the spray process is, that in nearly all cases the milk is partially condensed first. Among the roller-dried milks are Glaxo, Cow and Gate, Ambrosia. Spray-dried milks are Trufood, Milkall.

Most people find it difficult to memorise numbers and quantities when dealing with various feeding methods, and rely upon the instructions on the tin. These are fairly dependable in the best milks, but there is sometimes a tendency to make up solutions that are too strong. Roughly, most dried milks require diluting *eight times* to reconstitute ordinary milk, and this must be varied according to age, weight, digestion, etc.

Some firms sell a food which has dried milk as a basis with the addition of malted wheat in the place of extra lactose. Most of the best firms turn out, besides a simple dried milk, a " humanised " variety, which, by the additions of carbohydrates and fats, has been corrected to the appropriate percentage of human milk before the process of drying, and has also in some cases been subjected to an alteration of salts, e.g. the removal of some of the calcium and the addition of potassium salts. Reliable milks of this kind are : " Prescription," Glaxo, Allenbury's Food, Mead's Re-co-lac, Humanised Trufood.

Altogether, it may be said that the dried milks have a definite place in the feeding of infants. They are useful for children who are persistently intolerant of ordinary casein curds ; they can be used with advantage where the ordinary milk supply is really bad and the home conditions such as make the keeping of raw milk a difficult problem ; they may be used when weaning has to be carried out during the three hot months of the summer (July, August, September), while summer diarrhœa is prevalent ; they are invaluable for use while travelling.

On the other hand, dried milk has not proved itself superior to wet milk for the ordinary healthy child ; its use tends to an excessive fat formation, with its abundant evils ; the easy digestibility, while a welcome asset for the delicate child, is a snare and delusion in bringing up a healthy child and the education of its alimentary tract. The presence or absence of vitamines is still a debatable subject, and as long as vitamines can only be demonstrated qualitatively and quantitatively by biological tests, it will remain an open question whether " treated " milk can ever be as vital a food as the raw product.

Condensed Milk

Milk is condensed by being heated *in vacuo* for almost half an hour at the temperature of 100° Fahr., after preliminary pasteurisation at a temperature of about 150° Fahr. The result is a thick, creamy-looking substance which is not sterile, but has a comparatively low bacterial content when first manufactured. The process renders the proteins very readily digestible, but unfortunately destroys Vitamine C, and probably impairs both Vitamines A and B. Of reputable brands there are two varieties, the sweetened and unsweetened.

In sweetened condensed milk cane sugar has

been added, not only to bring the carbohydrate percentage up to that of human milk, but generally to a greater degree (as much as 20%), with the idea of rendering the milk comparatively free from bacteria. Tins of sweetened condensed milk last unsoured for several days after being opened.

Unsweetened condensed milk retains only its normal sugar content, and must be sweetened slightly if it is to be given to infants. It will not keep, once the tin is opened, any longer than ordinary milk.

There are a great many cheap varieties of condensed milk with a very poor nutritive value; many have been skimmed before condensing and have, therefore, a very low fat content, while their vitamine value is practically nil. Feeding on condensed milks for a prolonged period is fraught with danger, and the medical profession should make a definite stand against it. The habit is wide-spread, as condensed milk is cheap, easy to prepare, and often gives excellent immediate results, as it is readily digestible and often a rapid fat-former. It is sometimes even better tolerated than the mother's own milk, and is then a dreadful snare to the anxious mother who tries condensed milk feeding when she thinks her own milk " doesn't suit."

The ultimate effects of condensed milk are generally disastrous. The fat baby, who has flourished so well at first and put on a steady half-pound a week, gradually becomes pale, flabby, and irritable; he falls a victim to catarrhs of the respiratory and gastro-intestinal tracts, gets a large tympanitic belly, and finally shows in his bones all the signs of rickets. It is useless to quote the exceptions—the children we all meet with—who have flourished on condensed milk ; these are children with cast-iron constitutions, who would flourish on anything ! They make no difference to the general rule.

We must not, therefore, look upon condensed milk as being a satisfactory or adequate food for the period of infancy. We may, however, regard it as a really valuable help for temporary use in times of digestive disturbance. There are few modifications of milk so well tolerated, and it may be used as a temporary measure in many forms of digestive disturbance, during illness or after operations, in the early supplemental feeding of breast babies, and in cases of pylorospasm.

Other Modifications of Milk

Whey.—Before the term " humanised " was adopted by dried milk manufacturers, it was used almost exclusively for modifications of cow's milk and whey. The whey can be prepared by curdling cow's milk with rennet (either glycerinated preparations of rennet or rennet tablets). The curd removes the caseinogen and most of the fat, the whey containing all the sugar, the salts, and most of the lactalbumen ; if the curd be squeezed in a muslin bag some of the fat and casein return to the whey.

The whey is then used as a diluent of milk instead of water, and cream and lactose may be added to bring up the constituents to the percentages of human milk. The advantage of this method is that the infant can be accustomed gradually to the caseinogen of cow's milk by starting with whey only and having milk added in gradually increasing quantities.

The use of whey and sherry whey in diarrhœa is alluded to in the chapter on that subject.

Since Finkelstein's pronouncement that it was the whey, salts, and sugar of cow's milk which harmed the intestinal mucosa of the infant, rather than the protein curd, the use of whey has not been quite so popular, though much of his theory has been subsequently disproved.

Protein Milk.—Twenty years ago modification of cow's milk was all in the direction of cutting down the proteins, especially the casein, with the idea that infant dyspepsia was generally due to this constituent. Now that the prevailing theories blame fats and sugar for the majority of digestive disturbances, it is found advisable sometimes to add protein rather than reduce it, and to limit the fat and sugar constituents. Protein milk is generally made by the addition of some soluble protein, e.g. calcium caseinate, sold under the name of " Casec," to diluted milk, or even to skimmed milk where there is definite fat indigestion, and it may also be made with water only for cases of acute diarrhœa.

Prolonged feeding with protein milk should be avoided as the proteins cannot be adequately broken up without the presence of fat, and protein indigestion may result.

A preparation of lactalbumen, called Albulactin, is useful where extra protein is required. It may be added either to milk or whey according to circumstances. It should be borne in mind that lactalbumen is a more valuable protein than casein, especially for stimulating growth, as it contains a much larger proportion of cystin.

Acid Milk.—It has long been recognised that the salts of cow's milk differ very considerably from the salts of human milk, and that cow's milk requires a greater amount of hydrochloric acid than human milk before the hydrogen-ion concentration is great enough for peptic digestion to begin : the alkali " buffer " value of cow's milk is very high, that of dried or condensed milks rather lower, and that of human milk lowest of all. Unless, therefore, the infant's stomach can produce this increased amount of hydrochloric acid, gastric digestion of cow's milk will be deficient.

With this idea, hydrochloric acid may be added to milk (not the milk to the acid, or it will curdle), in the following proportions, given by Dr. Leonard Parsons : 2 drachms of decinormal hydrochloric acid and 2 drachms of water are added to each ounce of cow's milk. The milk does not curdle if it is fresh, and the mixture is taken well. Results have been good on the whole, though not startling. Citric acid may be used instead, ½ grain to the ounce of milk.

Lactic acid milk is sometimes given : 3 minims of the B.P. lactic acid to an ounce of milk.

Non-Milk Foods

Recently, a departure has been made from the practice of using milk as a basis for artificial feeding. A synthetic food called Almata has been introduced, and the manufacturers claim that it contains all necessary food elements in proper proportions for infant feeding. It is composed of egg-yolk, butter, malto-dextrins, maltose, salts, and de-citrated fruit juice. These constituents are made up into a fine yellow powder which is to be mixed with water only.

The idea of giving infants food which has no relation to milk (except for its butter constituent) is a comparatively new one. It is an interesting attempt and should certainly be given a trial, but it must be some time before really definite results can place its value in artificial feeding. It would be a useful food for the very few infants who from the first show a marked intolerance to any kind of milk.

Intervals between Feeds should be the same in artificial feeding as suggested for breast-feeding.

Amount of Food has also been mentioned in the chapter on breast-feeding. It is, however, impossible to lay down any fixed rules about amounts. It is best first to calculate how much milk an infant should be having in 24 hours, reckoning by its weight to start with, then modifying if the weight is out of proportion to the age (in either direction). The total amount may then be divided into the requisite number of feeds. Body weight alone is not a correct index; the extreme marasmic, weighing, perhaps, only 8 lb. at eight months old, requires and can digest a good deal more than the one pint of milk which his weight would suggest. Age alone is also not a correct index, or the fat two months old infant of 14 lb. would be getting too much.

To a certain extent the infant may judge for himself—but only to a certain extent. The baby who feeds very quickly has still got an appetite even when he has taken quite enough, and it is not well to give in to his hungry clamour and give him the extra ounce that he asks for. It must be remembered in this connection that over-feeding is a commoner fault than under-feeding, especially among the more well-to-do mothers.

On the other hand the sleepy premature cannot always be induced to take a sufficient quantity, and if he persistently refuses the amount which has been calculated as his due, smaller and more frequent feeds should be tried.

One thing that it is extremely difficult to impress upon mothers, even experienced ones, is that the hungry cry of a baby is very similar to the pain cry, and one has constantly to persuade them that what they take to be a demand for more food is often a cry due to flatulence or colic, and they are only increasing the trouble when they enlarge the feed.

The three indicators in prescribing an infant's diet are : (1) the weight chart ; (2) the condition of the stools ; (3) the general condition of the child, including its contentment and capacity for sleep. If these are satisfactory it is a temptation to let well alone, but it must be borne in mind that deficiency diseases develop slowly, and it is quite possible for a child taking condensed milk to be growing steadily in weight, passing well-digested stools, and appearing to flourish, while rickets is insidiously beginning to get a foothold ; so that it is only when these three indicators are satisfactory on a *theoretically adequate diet* that one's mind can be at rest.

CHAPTER V

FEEDING AFTER EARLY INFANCY

THE inexperienced medical officer is more at a loss when asked for advice about the feeding of small children, generally classed as " toddlers " at an Infant Welfare Centre, than when giving instructions for the feeding of infants. Destructive criticism is easy, but when it comes to constructing suitable dietaries for any given age, much care and thought are required. The most difficult period is before the end of the first year when milk still forms the bulk of the food, but other and more solid articles of diet are being introduced. The doctor who is going to have much to do with infants should first get a clear idea in his mind as to what food-stuffs are suitable for the young, and what they are likely to be able to digest at different ages ; he should also get some sort of practical idea as to the quantities that should be given. He should be able at a moment's notice to write down an alternative diet chart for any child under his care. Then, having made his own rules on the subject, he must be prepared to have them disregarded by the mother and flouted by the children. He will have to deal with every kind of individual, from the child who will eat anything as long as there is enough of it, to the child who fights against each new article of diet as it is introduced.

It is not always easy at the Clinic to find out exactly what a child is being fed on. The mothers know the right answers only too well, and, drawing on a vivid imagination, give a descripton of the child's meals which sounds a perfect model of correctness. Happily, the visiting nurse pays un-heralded calls and can given an ungarbled account of what she finds on the table.

As a practical point, milk should always be alluded to as " cow's milk " and butter as " real butter," otherwise condensed milk and margarine will be given.

SIX MONTHS TO ONE YEAR

There can be no absolute rule about the intro-duction of starchy foods. Babies who are having barley water as diluent are from an early age accustomed to a small percentage, and it is probable that from about the fourth month the pancreatic ferments are able to split it up into dextrin and maltose. It appears quite unnecessary to give starch earlier than the sixth or seventh month, and not even then if the child is breast-fed ; with the latter it is safe to wait till the ninth month if the child is progressing well. Indeed, it may be said that, in all the following suggestions, a breast-fed baby will generally be introduced to his foods rather later in age than a bottle-fed baby, partly because he does not take them so readily, and partly because a breast-fed child really does not seem to require the varied diet so soon as one which has been artificially fed.

The first introduction to this kind of food may be

in the form of a very milky cornflour or ground-rice mixture or thin groats. The usual mistake is to give too much, and to expect the child to consume a whole saucerful at a meal. If one to two table-spoonfuls are taken before the midday bottle or breast feed, that will be quite sufficient at first. Later, when the child has got accustomed to a thickened milk feed, he may be given something a little more solid in the shape of rusk and milk. A rusk may be halved; one half is given to the baby to chew, which he is more than willing to do as his teeth are coming through and he is already thrusting anything he can reach into his mouth. The hard rusk is soothing to bite on, and when soaked with saliva crumbles up finely and is not likely to break off in lumps and choke the child, as a crust of bread may do. The other half of the rusk is soaked in milk and given for the midday meal. *Five feeds* a day are still being given, and as the starchy part of the midday meal is increased, a few ounces may be omitted from the bottle that follows. In the case of the breast-fed child, the cornflour or rusk feed is probably his first introduc-tion to cow's milk, and as it is different from his accustomed diet he will often want a great deal of persuading before he will take it. Many mothers prefer to wean the baby on to a bottle before attempting the starchy feed.

Fruit juice, e.g. that of orange or grape, can be given at a very early age, and is frequently used for artificially fed babies to prevent scurvy. Very little is required, two to three teaspoonfuls of sweetened orange juice being ample for one day. It is not always easily borne, and may cause colic.

From about nine months old the pulp of fruit may be used in moderation, both for its anti-scorbutic and laxative actions. For this purpose a tablespoonful of well-mashed baked or stewed apple may be given two or three times a week.

Egg may be introduced at the ninth or tenth month. Only the yolk should be used at first, and bearing in mind that it is a highly concentrated, fatty food only very little must be given at a time ; half a yolk with some of the rusk and followed by 6 ounces of milk, will make a good meal, and should be limited to two or three times a week. Egg may also be used now in the form of custard, either baked or boiled.

Eggs should always be specifically mentioned when giving instructions to mothers about custards, otherwise they may use artificial custard powders, the cheaper of which contain no eggs at all.

Potato may be used if old floury potatoes are available ; they must be well cooked and may be mashed up with a little butter. They can be given with milk, but to make a change it is advisable to add a little fresh meat juice or gravy occasionally, or, alternatively, they may be soaked in chicken or mutton broth. Other vegetables are, perhaps, better left until a later period.

By the end of the first year, milk is still the main part of the food and should be taken exclusively in the early morning and late evening feed ; the three feeds in the middle of the day may be varied with simple foods as suggested above, and the total amount of milk taken should have been decreased to about a pint and a half.

A Year Old

Up till now there have been five feeds a day, but after the first twelve months the healthy, flourishing baby should begin to think about dropping the late evening bottle. Happily, many of them drop it themselves ; they are put to sleep after a good feed at 6 p.m., and scarcely wake again until the early morning hours ; or they wake up at 10 to have the bottle and fall asleep again before more than a few ounces are taken. Others are more difficult to break of the habit, and in those many unfortunate cases where the whole family lives in one room, the baby is almost certain to wake for a 10 o'clock feed for many months after it should be sleeping the night through. There is no necessity to cut off this evening feed suddenly—it is better to reduce it in amount quite gradually, till it becomes merely a little drink.

That reduces the meals to four a day, and they must correspondingly be made a little bigger. Here it must be remembered that the sleeping habits of babies of the poorer classes must necessarily be quite different from those of the well-to-do. Our own babies are asleep between 6 and 7 in the evening, and often awake at the ungodly hour of 5.30 ; they are quite ready for a feed by 6 a.m. and will some-times, but not always, sleep again. The poor baby of the same age (between 1 and 2 years) has often had a snatch of sleep at 6 p.m., but wakes up again when father and the family come in and does not really settle down for the night until nearly 10 o'clock ; consequently he often sleeps until 8 a.m. The Clinic doctor should take this into account when giving advice about the number and time of meals.

Bread should not be given too early, as it forms a glutinous mass, and is by no means so easy to digest as rusks and biscuits. Of necessity it forms a great part of the diet of the poorer classes, and often too large a proportion when the mother is too busy or too ignorant to vary the carbohydrate supply with puddings. The chief point to insist on is that the bread should be stale, and this is a point that really needs driving home, as stale bread is rarely seen in poor homes ; educated mothers would be horrified to see the newness of the bread that is given to the infants in the slums. Wholemeal bread should be frequently used alternately with white bread, especially for children who have a tendency to constipation. Unfortunately they do not often like it.

Butter is a valuable food and should always be supplied to children when the family means can run to it. At a year old the baby may be given a few fingers of bread-and-butter at his 8 to 8.30 a.m meal and again at tea-time.

Margarine, which is generally made from vegetable fats, is moderately nutritive, but does not possess nearly such a high anti-rachitic value as butter. It is, of course, better than no fat at all.

Dripping is a useful fat food, and may often be given on bread to save the butter.

Milk.—There is a very common tendency during the second year of life for a child to grow tired of milk. It is so common that one cannot help wondering whether it is not a natural phenomenon, and whether one should not take it as an indication that milk is not really required in large quantities after the first year of life. Very few children, when they come to the cup stage of feeding, take plain milk with pleasure, even though they have consumed it exclusively for months beforehand from the bottle. They drink a certain amount because they are thirsty, but they would prefer water.

The consequence is, that either milk is given up altogether—the usual result with those who can ill afford it—or it has to be coaxed down by disguising with cocoa or tea. In families where fresh butter, eggs, good meat, and vegetables are easily obtained, the milk fetish may well be given up if the child turns against it, but not, of course, until a full varied diet has been established.

But in circles where stews, tinned salmon, and margarine prevail it is, perhaps, as well to insist on the use of milk for children as long as possible. Cocoa makes milk more interesting, but it must be made thin, as its fat globules are coarse and not too easily tolerated. Sweetened tea is even more popular, and here one is confronted with a problem. Shall one allow the " dash of tea " that makes milk bearable as a drink to the average child, or ought one to put off as long as possible the introduction of a beverage which, taken strong and often, annually ruins thousands of digestions ? This question can only be answered by considering in each individual case whether the milk is really such an important part of the diet that it must, at this cost, be made palatable.

Water.—Children, wise people, always want water at odd times between meals, and as it is far better for them to drink then than at meals, the usual cry of " I want a drink o' water," should never be disregarded. Mothers should be advised not to forget water for the infant who cannot yet ask.

Milk Puddings may be started very early and are graduated from the thin floury paste given to the newly weaned baby to the more solid rice, tapioca, semolina puddings, and cornflour shapes given to the older child. They are an excellent way of giving milk and well-cooked starch, and young children generally take them well.

Suet puddings should be started later, not till about two years old.

Pastries and new buns are a perfect pest. Very few Clinic mothers will admit that they give them to their children, but it is a common sight to see a pram standing outside a shop with two or three small children munching horrible-looking confections while the mother does her shopping in peace.

Vegetables, both greens and roots, are valuable for their vegetable protein, cellulose, salts, and vitamines. They are comparatively inexpensive, and should be used freely in the child's diet. The dislike for vegetables so often shown by young children is probably often due to the fact that their mothers cook them so badly. Of late years there has been a great vogue for uncooked vegetables, and one often hears that people are advised to give raw carrots, etc., to the young, presumably with the idea that uncooked vegetables retain their vitamines and salts unchanged in a way that is impossible with the cooked article. Vitamines and salts are of no value, however, unless they can be used, and it must be remembered that raw vegetables are very difficult things to digest. It is not uncommon to find pieces of unaltered carrot in the fæces of a child even when they have been cooked. How much more likely is the raw vegetable to pass through undigested !

Fruit should always be used for children when it can be procured, but it is, unfortunately, expensive for needy families. Apples should be given, baked or stewed, up to eighteen months old, and after that they may alternatively be given raw ; but they must be ripe. A ghastly thing called a " toffee-apple," beloved of small boys, is a green, unripe apple dipped into toffee and impaled on a stick. Bananas may be given even during the first year, provided they are quite ripe and are well-mashed into a pulp, but a very small child given a whole banana in its fist will generally swallow large lumps which may cause considerable trouble. Oranges are useful ; at first the juice only, then juice and pulp, and finally the membranous part as well. Grapes also are very good for children.

Uncooked stone fruits of all kinds (dried prunes excepted) are undesirable on the whole. Perhaps there is nothing specifically deleterious in them, but it is difficult to get such quickly ripening fruit at exactly the right stage, and they are either given unripe, when they cause colic, or over-ripe, when they cause diarrhœa. The same may be said for fresh fruit such as gooseberries, raspberries, currants and strawberries.

Meat may be introduced at about eighteen months and should at first be minced. Beef, mutton, chicken, or rabbit may be used. Only a little should be given and by no means every day. Later, the child may be encouraged to masticate by being given cut-up meat rather than minced meat.

Fish should be boiled or preferably steamed, and not fried. Unfortunately, fried fish and chips from the shop round the corner is such a convenient dish that it generally finds its way early into the diet of the slum child, and soon gives him a distaste for anything so insipid as steamed fish ; dried and salted fish and tinned salmon do the same.

CHAPTER VI

NORMAL STOOLS: CONSTIPATION

A PRACTICAL acquaintance with the character of infants' stools is indispensable to the Welfare Medical Officer, and he must especially familiarise himself with the wide variations in the stools passed by normal babies. Mothers should be encouraged to display the last soiled napkin, as their own descriptions are apt to be incorrect and misleading.

After the meconium has been passed (during the first few days after birth), the breast-fed child should produce a bright yellow, homogeneous stool, semi-solid, but quite unformed, and with a clean acid smell. One to three stools a day are passed, the total amount being roughly 1 to 3% of the amount of food taken, the proportion being slightly larger during the first two to three weeks.

So long as the amount is sufficient it matters very little whether there are one, two, or three actions. Any number greater than three suggests a too rapid peristalsis and insufficient absorption.

The bottle-fed baby generally has a stool of a rather different character. The colour, instead of being canary yellow, tends to be pale ; this is due to the greater reduction and decomposition of bile pigments which takes place during digestion of cow's milk. The bulk, also, is greater as there is more residue, so that a sluggish intestinal action may lead to the passage of a formed mass even in a quite young infant.

After the first few weeks the digestive mechanism of the infant will get into an automatic action if its daily routine is kept even and undisturbed. When feeds, outings, and sleeps can be kept to the same hours every day, the tendency is for the bowels also to act regularly at the same times. The infant will normally have a motion after its first morning feed, as the gastro-colic reflex will naturally be more active after some hours of fasting. The habit of passing an early morning stool is a beneficial one, and the natural inclination should be encouraged from the first by holding the baby on a small receptacle directly after the first feed. This may be done from about four weeks of age, and it is wonderful how quickly young infants learn to take the hint. Mothers too will soon find that there is less waste of time in doing this than in washing out soiled napkins.

It cannot be repeated too often to mothers, individually and collectively, that establishing good habits in connection with defæcation, and maintaining those habits through childhood, will do much to keep their children in good health and prevent one of the commonest of modern curses—constipation. Many mothers are more or less careful with infants during the first few years of life, but once the children start going to school have only the vaguest idea of their daily habits, and try to make up for their ignorance during the week by administering an aperient to the whole family on Saturday night. This weekly dose is almost a religion among the uneducated classes ; it is a pernicious habit, but one

can understand that a busy working woman finds
it difficult to superintend five or six children in
this respect, and feels it to be her duty to make
certain of at least one good action a week. Children
should use the bedroom article on the floor as long
as possible, the position of defæcation being then a
squatting one, with thighs well flexed. When
they have perforce to take to the lavatory seat, they
should be made to rest the feet firmly on a stool in
front of them ; the position of sitting with hanging
legs is always bad, defæcation is more difficult, and
herniæ may be produced from lack of support of the
abdominal walls.

VARIATIONS

Retention of Fæces.—This is an extremely common
fault in young infants up to about three months old.
It occurs most frequently in the fat, lethargic baby
who is a big feeder and a good sleeper. Intestinal
peristalsis is perfectly good up to a point, but the
rectal reflex is sluggish. The well-digested fæces
collect in the lower part of the colon, but often
seem to cause little or no discomfort; the afferent
impulses to the cord are sluggish and the emptying
reflex simply fails to take place. The child may
fail to pass a motion for forty-eight hours or more.
Usually it is uncomfortable and fretful after a time,
and suffers from flatulence, but sometimes there
seems to be no discomfort at all. The mother
calls this condition " constipation," and seeks to
relieve the child with purgatives. One should
immediately suspect the diagnosis of " constipation "
in any child under three months old, and the first
question should be, " Is the motion soft and fluid

when the baby does pass it at last ? " It nearly always is, and one can proceed to explain to the mother that it is " laziness," not constipation, and the child is in no need of purgatives, which merely irritate a perfectly good, active stomach and intestine.

There are some who advise leaving the condition alone, and allowing the infant its forty-eight or even seventy-two hours interval between evacuations. This may be a sound policy when no discomfort is evidenced ; but discomfort and restlessness usually develop, and may be easily relieved by the introduction of a small glycerine suppository into the rectum. The suppository should be the smallest (infant) size. It is not chosen for the hygroscopic property of the glycerine, for the glycerine has no time to act as such. It is chosen because it is soft and pliable, easily introduced, not at all likely to injure the mucous membrane of the rectum, and yet a large enough foreign body to cause an active stimulation of the rectal emptying reflex. Soap is sometimes used, but it is not easy to make a soap suppository soft enough to be harmless to the mucous membrane.

The suppository should be moistened with water or smeared with vaseline, and introduced into the rectum with the little finger. Usually within thirty seconds the contents of the rectum and sigmoid colon have been completely turned out.

True Constipation.—When the motion is formed and infrequent true constipation may be said to exist. In young infants on the breast the commonest cause is an insufficient supply of milk, and in these cases particular attention should be paid to the mother's diet, etc. (see Chapter III). Water should be given freely between feeds, and, if necessary, supplementary feeding adopted. Over-feeding is occasionally a cause of constipation. The stool is then rather massive, formed, and often offensive. It is not passed easily owing to its bulk. Thirdly, an important though happily not a frequent cause of constipation is hypertrophic pyloric stenosis. Vomiting combined with constipation in a breast-fed baby during the early weeks of life should always suggest this condition and lead to a careful examination for the pyloric tumour and peristaltic wave. In *bottle-fed babies* an investigation of the causes of true constipation must include not only the amount of food being given, but the quality and quantity of the different food elements.

Fat.—It was formerly thought that a deficiency of fat in the food was a cause of constipation, but it has been found that in many cases the stools of a constipated infant contain much soap, fatty acid and neutral fats, and opinion is rather tending towards considering excess of fat a cause of constipation. Certainly a deficiency of bile leads to sluggish peristalsis ; and without bile the fat is not able to be well assimilated. In this connection it may be mentioned that well-to-do mothers often choose " top " milk for their infants, thereby giving them a much higher percentage of fat than is desirable if they are taking " whole milk " ; even if diluted feeds are being given it is an unscientific and inexact way of adding cream.

Protein Curds.—Much that is contradictory is written about the place of casein in causation of the constipation of infants. It is sometimes said that an excess of casein produces a massive dry stool which is passed with difficulty. On the other hand, it is known that a large stool stimulates peristalsis so much better than a small one. If the latter is true, a big residue of casein curd should lead to free action of the bowels.

Actually, it is found that the infant weaned from the breast to raw milk frequently becomes constipated. Possibly this condition has nothing to do with casein, but depends on the difference in salts, especially excess of calcium in cow's milk.

Carbohydrates.—As fermentation of sugars stimulates peristalsis, it is possible that food with too little carbohydrate may cause constipation. The sugars have different values in this respect ; perhaps the most useful is maltose.

Organic Disease, such as obstruction at any part of the intestine or rectum or the presence of megacolon, need not be enlarged upon here, but must be borne in mind as possible though rare causes of constipation in infancy.

Treatment

Water.—It is most important that the daily fluid intake should be adequate, and all babies, breast-fed or artificially fed, should have plain water feeds occasionally (say 2 to 4 ozs. twice a day, according to age). The taking of extra water will not cure obstinate constipation as a rule, but the regular habit may prevent it.

If the stool has a fatty appearance, fat in the food should be reduced ; this proceeding is often effectual.

Extra carbohydrates, especially maltose, are often

most successful in curing constipation in young bottle-fed infants. Maltose may be added to each feed (about 3½ to 3j), or Mellin's may be given in the milk (this is chiefly malto-dextrin).

Fruit juice, e.g. orange or grape, is frequently advised for bottle-fed babies. It is chiefly used as an anti-scorbutic, but it has a mildly laxative action and may be given if it does not cause colic.

Massage of the abdomen may be practised, but is rather dangerous in unskilled hands.

Purgatives.—When everything has been done in the way of modifying the quantity and quality of the food, there still remains a large number of cases in which some form of aperient must be used. Before prescribing even the mildest of drugs for chronic constipation it is advisable to explain to the mother how and why they are to be given. She should be told that the medicine is not to be given occasionally to produce a purging action, but must be given constantly in small doses. Often she will have to regulate the dose herself, and she must by careful observation discover the amount necessary to produce a good daily action without purging the child. It should be explained to her that her aim is to get the bowels into a regular daily habit, and that once the habit is formed it may be possible to lessen the dose gradually and finally abandon the drug altogether.

Liquid Paraffin is frequently used in doses of 3j given one to four times daily ; it acts as a lubricant and partly also as an intestinal stimulant. It is successful in mild cases of constipation, but has certain drawbacks. As the intestine learns to tolerate the paraffin the dose has to be increased,

and since this happens early in many cases it has
to be abandoned, as it is inadvisable to give very large
doses. It is suggested by some that the paraffin
forms a thin coat over the mucous membrane and
when spread over a large area may interfere seriously
with the absorption of food. This is theoretically
true, but no exact observations have been published
and it is not generally found that babies tend to
waste when taking liquid paraffin.

Recently, various compounds have been prepared
of paraffin with malt (e.g. Cristolax), paraffin
with agar (e.g. Petrolagar), many of them excellent preparations for those who can afford
them, but rather beyond the purses of the Welfare
mothers.

Mercury in the form of Hydrargyrum cum Creta
is a useful drug in infancy. As an aperient it
may be given in doses of $\frac{1}{8}$ to $\frac{1}{4}$ grain three times
daily, but, as with other aperients, the individual
reaction varies so much that the dose appropriate
to each child can only be found by experiment.
If purging is avoided the preparation may be given
for quite long periods without harmful consequences,
though of course the sooner it can be diminished
and abandoned the better.

Phenolphthalein in doses of a $\frac{1}{2}$ to 1 grain is a
mild aperient, causing little or no griping ; it has
been used for children during the last twenty years,
and is generally successful. This drug has many
proprietary pseudonyms, of which " Purgen " is
perhaps the best known.

Compound Syrup of Figs, though generally kept
for older children, may be used for infants if milder
remedies have failed. This compound contains

senna among other ingredients, and is a fairly strong aperient. Infants should be started with a half-teaspoonful at night, and the dose varied according to the result.

Castor Oil has no place in the treatment of chronic constipation. It is useful as a single purge at the onset of any illness, for colic due to an error of diet, or in the early stages of acute diarrhœa, but its action is too vigorous, and being generally followed by a decrease in peristalsis and consequent paralysis of the bowel, it is to be avoided in these cases of intestinal stasis.

Olive Oil acts as an aperient in very young infants, who, however, rarely suffer from true constipation. It should not be used for mere retention of fæces. Very soon the child is too old for it.

Constipation after Infancy

Between the ages of two and five a number of children develop a habit of constipation, even when they have been perfectly regular and normal as infants. They do not always show any ill effects at first, but after a time they develop fretfulness, loss of appetite, sleeplessness and pallor, and occasionally loss of weight. Constipation is so frequently associated with chronic gastritis and furred tongue that it is difficult to know which started first. In many cases the mother's carelessness with regard to the child's daily habits may be to blame, or there may be lack of fresh air and exercise, or the diet may be insufficient in quantity or deficient in quality. The constipation may start when the child, enfeebled during convalescence from whooping cough, measles, or some other illness, forms a bad habit, which persists even when the body has recovered tone.

There are also many cases of constipation in children whose training, diet, etc., seem to be beyond reproach.

Diet.—This should be carefully regulated. It is often found that there has been a large preponderance of starch and sugars, with too little protein and fat, and very little cellulose. Wholemeal bread and oatmeal should replace white bread ; vegetables and fruit may be used freely ; plenty of water should be given to drink, and the appetite for meals must not be impaired by the constant sucking of sweets and eating of buns at odd times.

Daily exercise in the open air is important, but unfortunately difficult for the Welfare mother to manage, especially when the child has left the pram stage but is not yet old enough to be allowed out by itself.

When school age is reached, the hurried breakfast and early start militate against the continuance of healthy habits ; and when one considers that in many houses there is one w.c. to be shared by four families, it is not surprising that children rush off to school in the morning without waiting to relieve themselves.

Drugs.—These should be used when necessary in the same manner as described for infants. The weekly purge must be avoided, and whatever preparation is used should be calculated to produce one or two motions a day without griping pains.

Syrup of figs, liquorice powder, senna, cascara, aloin, phenolphthalein, rhubarb, may be prescribed alone or in some combination.

6

CHAPTER VII

ABNORMAL STOOLS : DIARRHŒA

Acid Stools

THE reaction of stools of the breast-fed baby is slightly acid ; it is usually neutral in bottle feeding. Any marked increase in acidity is due to digestive disturbances of the upper part of the intestine, and in the case of artificial feeding is generally caused by excessive fermentation of the sugar content of the milk. The stools may be frothy or may look quite normal. The nates are reddened, however quickly the diaper is changed, and if the condition continues they rapidly become excoriated. The treatment is simple and quickly efficacious. Carbohydrates should be cut down, and soothing ointment applied to the buttocks :

R Olei Ricini   .   .   .   . ʒij
   Unguenti Zinci .   .   .   . ℥j
   Unguenti Acidi Borici   .   . ℥j

Alkaline Stools

Alkaline Stools are due either to Protein indigestion or catarrh of the large bowel. In the latter case there is an excess of mucus in the stool, and occasionally a little blood. This condition also excoriates the skin, and sometimes leaves little round punched-out ulcers which are sluggish and heal with difficulty. *Treatment.*—Cause 1. Decrease the protein element of the food, especially casein. Cause 2. Wash out the colon and give bismuth.

CURDY STOOLS

The whitish or pale-yellow lumps and flakes seen in the stool are composed sometimes of fat, sometimes of protein, more often the former. They are rarely pure, and, while ether will dissolve most of a fat curd, a little insoluble protein is often found with it, and conversely a curd which is chiefly composed of protein may stain with Sudan ii.

FAT CURDS

The fat-splitting ferment of the pancreas is not well developed in early life, so that it is not surprising if a certain proportion of fat fails to be digested, and that that portion appears in the stools as often in the form of neutral fat as of fatty acids or soaps. There is at first considerable difficulty with cow's cream, as the fat globules are far coarser than those of human milk fat. For this reason, when a child is being weaned from the breast to cow's milk, the accurate percentage of fat should not be given until a tolerance to this kind of fat has been established. An unusual degree of fat indigestion, occurring during the second or third year, would suggest cœliac disease.

Treatment.—Fatty stools rapidly lead to diarrhœa, wasting, etc. It is better at first to give feeds entirely free from fat, i.e. skimmed milk, and to add fat cautiously after a few days. It is sometimes advisable to change the kind of fat for a little while. For example, a child getting fat indigestion on ordinary milk may be given skimmed milk and cod liver oil, or skimmed milk and Virol for a change.

Protein Curds

Cow's milk, with its considerable excess of caseinogen over lactalbumen, is curdled by the action of acid and rennin into a tough clot, the caseinogen being thrown out of its colloid state. Human milk only forms a very fine, flocculent curd, and it is supposed that this *equal* quantity of lactalbumen keeps the caseinogen of human milk in its colloid form. In the same way such substances as starch, dextrin, and malto-dextrin may exert this influence on caseinogen and keep it from forming such a solid, thick clot in the stomach. Hence the rationale of the various preparations of malted wheats for infants' foods.

Feeding by untreated raw milk is therefore likely to lead to curd indigestion until toleration has been established. Even when the milk has been mixed with barley water or with dextrins, or treated with citrate of soda, curds may find their way into the stools and may set up diarrhœa.

Curds, both acid and fat, may be present to a small extent in the motions consistent with steady gain in weight and lack of discomfort. Babies who habitually take large feeds sometimes pass curds, and they are present when intestinal peristalsis is too energetic and motions frequent. Their presence should, however, always be regarded with suspicion, and measures taken to prevent them.

GREEN STOOLS

Stools may vary from a yellowish-green tinge to a bright spinach green. Probably the colour is due to oxidation of the normal bilirubin which generally colours the infant's stools, but Lesage considers that it may sometimes be due to the growth of special chromogenetic bacteria (not *b. pyocyaneus*) in the fæces. Sometimes a stool, though yellow when passed, turns green on exposure to the air; in this case it is almost certainly oxidation of bilirubin. Occasionally breast-fed babies have green stools; these are passed frequently, generally one after each feed. The child is generally being over-fed or fed too quickly.

MUCOUS STOOLS

Excess of mucus in the stools indicates catarrh of the colon. This may be brought about by unsuitable feeding and diarrhœa, or may be the result of constipation. In the latter case it is a protective phenomenon. When the inflammation of the colon is excessive blood may be mixed with the mucus.

When constipation is the cause treatment should be towards softening and liquefying the stool. When the colitis is part of a general diarrhœa bismuth and small doses of grey powder may be given, and the colon may be gently irrigated with plain water.

BLOOD IN THE STOOLS

Blood in the stools may occur: (1) in acute colitis (as above); (2) from a rectal polypus; in this case the stool is generally normal, without mucus, and the blood is bright ; (3) when there is intussusception of the bowel : this is a very serious accident, but happily not often difficult to diagnose : the symptoms of sudden screams of pain, vomiting, malæna, and rapid collapse are striking in a hitherto healthy child, and the sausage-shaped tumour can generally be felt ; (4) in purpura hæmorrhagica, when there are signs of bleeding elsewhere.

Offensive Stools

The fæces pass through the gastro-intestinal tract more quickly in infants than in adults, and there is not much time for putrefactive processes to take place. There is, therefore, very little disagreeable smell about the healthy infant's fæces.

The stools of a breast-fed child have a faintly acid smell, very distinctive. The sour smell is sometimes exaggerated when the growth of lactic acid organisms is very active. A more distinctively fæcal smell occurs when the colon group of bacilli are causing putrefaction, especially when peristalsis is slow and the fæces get held up. In later childhood an offensive-smelling stool is generally associated with exaggerated putrefactive processes, and it is sometimes found that too much meat is being given.

Diarrhœa

The term diarrhœa is very vaguely used, but should properly only apply when the stools are markedly increased in number. The condition is generally associated with indigestion and with abnormality of stools such as those above mentioned, there being usually a combination of various conditions, a motion, for instance, being curdy, green, and mixed with mucus at the same time. It should be understood, however, that, though diarrhœa is generally a secondary condition, dependent on the abnormalities of digestion, it may in some cases be primary (e.g. when caused by acute infection), and the undigested stool merely a product of too rapid peristalsis.

The causes of diarrhœa in infants may, then, be classed as :

1. Faults in Diet.
2. Infection of the stomach and intestines.
3. Tuberculosis.
4. Cœliac diseases (pathogenesis unknown).

The first cause accounts for a very large majority of the cases, and has been discussed under the heading of Abnormal Stools. The quality of the stool is the important point, and the number of stools is not often greatly increased, especially if the onset has not been rapid. This form of diarrhœa can best be treated by careful dieting after due attention to the character of the stools. It is helpful to start the case with a partial starvation diet for 24 hours, consisting of water, albumen water, and half-strength normal saline ; this last, if sweetened, does not taste at all disagreeable, and is usually taken very well. This must not be kept up too long, as the baby is rarely in a state to stand much abstention from food. The colon may be washed out the first day. The subsequent feeding depends entirely on the variety of indigestion as demonstrated in the stools.

Sometimes it is advisable to change the type of food altogether for the time being. For instance, an infant who has been having a raw milk mixture may be put on to unsweetened condensed milk for a few weeks, or dried milk may be changed to raw milk plus a malted wheat. Subsequently, the original feeding may be reverted to if it had hitherto been satisfactory.

Drugs are of very little value in this type of diarrhœa. Calomel and grey powder seem to be useful at times when given in very small doses, though their action is uncertain. Calomel gr. $\frac{1}{10}$ or hyd. c̄ cret. gr. $\frac{1}{8}$ given two or three times a day.

Acute Infection of the Gastro-Intestinal Tract

This occurs epidemically during the summer months, from about mid-July till the end of September, the onset of the epidemic depending on the ground temperature, and generally starting rather abruptly when the temperature of the earth at 4 ft. deep = 56° Fahr.

No single specific organism has been discovered; bacteriological investigations show that numerous and varied flora may be present in the stools; these include *Shiga bacillus*, *Flexner Harris b.*, *Morgan's b.*, *b. enteritidis of Gaertner*, and *b. paratyphosus (B.)* Contaminated milk is thought to be a common cause of infection, but the disease is also directly infectious, and can spread rapidly through the children's ward of a hospital even under the best conditions. Flies are suspected as carriers. Ideally, these cases should be isolated as rigorously as scarlet-fever and diphtheria, but this is rarely practicable. During a hot summer there are many thousands of cases in every large town, and the mortality is high. Recently, doubts have been expressed as to the bacterial origin of summer diarrhœa, but up to the present no better explanation has been forthcoming, and although it is true that the pathogenic organisms present are various, the clinical nature of the disease and its epidemiological characters are much in favour of its being an infection, probably a specific one.

Symptoms.—Acute gastro-enteritis by no means confines itself to the feeble and wasting. Healthy looking, well-nourished babies are frequently attacked. Breast-fed babies are not altogether exempt, though the incidence among them is low, and the type of attack not as a rule so serious. The onset may be very sudden, and the first symptom is generally *vomiting*. The vomiting is more or less violent and frequent for two or three days; after this it stops altogether in the majority of cases, but persists in some for a week or more. The *diarrhœa* sets in soon after the onset, and becomes rapidly worse, until by the third day the infant may be passing ten to fifteen stools a day. These are fluid, green, offensive, and flaked with curds and mucus. The *temperature* is usually raised at first, sometimes as high as 104° Fahr., but some cases are apyrexial from the first. The *pulse* is quick and feeble. *Wasting* is astonishingly rapid, and the skin becomes inelastic. *Convulsions* may occur at any time in the course of an attack. In severe cases death may occur within a few days of the onset. Even in favourable cases recovery is always slow, and it may be weeks or even months before the child passes a natural stool again.

The most depressing cases, and they are very frequent, are those in which the child survives the acute febrile stage, retains its hold on life for a week or two, then collapses and dies just when its chances are beginning to appear hopeful.

Prevention should be constantly preached in the Welfare Centre, especially from June onwards. Occasional short talks to the mothers on the subject of cleaning jugs, boiling bottles, covering milk, and slaughtering flies, might be given with advantage. Soiled napkins should be placed immediately in a covered pail full of water, and preferably a little disinfectant, such as Lysol, added. At the Welfare Centre an attempt should be made to keep diarrhœa cases apart from healthy babies. Properly, these babies should be attending a private doctor or hospital clinic, but during the summer months they appear in large numbers at Welfare Clinics and are often mixed indiscriminately with healthy babies.

Treatment.—At the start a dose of castor oil should be given, though this is by no means always retained, and all milk stopped. The diet for the first 24 or 48 hours may consist of plain water, albumen water, or half-strength normal saline solution slightly sweetened. Brandy is very useful, and may be given in four-hourly doses of m. x to m.xxx, according to age. The principal problem is to keep enough fluid in the child's tissues, which are constantly depleted by vomiting and diarrhœa. *Intra-venous* injections are only possible in young infants by the drastic proceeding of cutting down on to the veins. The wounds heal with difficulty.

Sub-cutaneous injections are slowly absorbed, but

they are not satisfactory, and puncture wounds often become septic even when the utmost care has been used. *Rectal* injections are generally useless, as they are quickly returned. *Intra-peritoneal* injections are absorbed well, and are satisfactory on the whole, but some risk of bowel perforation attends their administration.

Intestinal Antiseptics are rather disappointing, as it is generally impossible to give a drug in such strength that it is sufficient to kill morbid bacteria without damaging the tissues. Various synthetic compounds have been brought forward, most of them based on a phenol derivative, e.g. dimol, kerol, etc. ; Guaiacol and beta-naphthol have also been used. Some observers claim a certain amount of success with these drugs, but the results cannot be said to be striking. Preparations of lactic acid bacteria are sometimes given, as their growth is said to inhibit the growth of putrefactive and other organisms ; this is certainly the case *in vitro*, but the action may not be quite the same *in vivo*.

Some kind of food should be given as soon as possible ; it is unwise to keep these babies too long on water only. A good beginning is to give whey or sherry whey. The latter is prepared by adding 5 oz. of cooking sherry to a pint of milk, and straining off the resulting curd. The whey contains lactalbumen, lactose, salts, a very little fat, water, and alcohol. It is, however, an inexact way of giving alcohol and often too much is given. It is better as a rule to give whey prepared by the ordinary method and add brandy as required. After 24 or 48 hours of whey feeds, a little milk may be added, or a protein feed may be given for a short time.

Few cases have a straightforward course, and it is often necessary to go right back to the first step of water only, whenever a relapse occurs.

Acute and rapidly collapsing cases are best nursed in a hospital, as the preliminary treatment cannot be carried out satisfactorily in the ordinary home ; but it is a mistake to keep them too long. They should be taken home directly they are on the upward path, for it is a fact, rather difficult to explain, that relapses occur more often in babies who are kept in the ward in a convalescent stage than in those sent to their homes, however poor, crowded, and insanitary those homes may be.

Abdominal Tuberculosis

This is not by any means a common cause of diarrhœa in infants under two years old, though the expression " consumptive bowels " is such a commonplace among the Clinic mothers that one could imagine it to be of frequent occurrence. The diagnosis is either their own or that of a kindly doctor who has wished to supply a good-sounding title for a mere error in diet.

From about two years old onwards abdominal tuberculosis may make its appearance in varying forms. Those cases in which free fluid is present in the peritoneal cavity and those in which tuberculous masses may be felt present little difficulty in diagnosis, but there is a large group of cases where the infection probably never gets beyond the mesenteric glands. In these the symptoms and signs are not very definite : there is general wasting ; some enlargement of the abdomen, with a tympanitic percussion note and the feeling which has been well described as " doughy " ; liver and spleen may both be bulky ; there may be slight evening pyrexia, and diarrhœa often alternates with periods of constipation. As the foregoing is also a faithful picture of the condition brought about by prolonged dietetic errors, and as both classes of case do very well on hospital or convalescent home treatment with regular dieting, fresh air, and general hygienic measures, it will be seen that the diagnosis of tuberculous abdominal glands or early tuberculous peritonitis frequently remains in doubt.

CŒLIAC DISEASE

Cœliac Disease is still little understood. It is a chronic form of diarrhœa, the stools being large, pale, offensive, and containing an undue proportion of fats (neutral, fatty acids, and soaps). The condition often leads to infantilism, but is sometimes recovered from completely. A detailed account of the condition and the various theories of its causation may be found in medical textbooks.

CHAPTER VIII

VOMITING

THE symptom of vomiting occurs with great frequency in all childish complaints and illnesses. Children vomit with very little effort and often with no discomfort. The small boy who has eaten too many jam tarts wakes in the middle of the night, completely rejects the contents of his stomach, and five minutes afterwards is sleeping the sleep of the innocent. The ability to get rid of any noxious material from the stomach is a most valuable asset of childhood, and saves a lot of trouble for the rest of the digestive apparatus.

A large majority of cases of vomiting depend upon some temporary cause (dietetic), or some active local damage, e.g. gastritis. At the same time one must always be on the look out for other morbid conditions, as central vomiting and reflex vomiting are common enough symptoms in many of the diseases of childhood.

The vomiting of infancy may be considered under the following headings :

Overflow

Gastric irritation
$\begin{cases} \text{temperature of food} \\ \text{bulk of food} \\ \text{quality of food} \end{cases}$
$\begin{cases} \text{excess of fat} \\ \text{large curds} \\ \text{impurities} \end{cases}$

Gastritis
Constipation

Congenital Hypertrophic Pyloric Stenosis
Pylorospasm
Nervous
Cerebral
Symptomatic

OVERFLOW

Infants share with some of their elders an inability to gauge the capacity of their stomachs, and a healthy, hungry babe frequently takes more at a feed than it can properly deal with. Happily at this early age the remedy is automatic, and the stomach duly returns the surplus. This overflow at the end of a meal is generally referred to by the mothers as " healthy " or " natural " vomiting. The baby should, however, be discouraged from over-filling itself, as it gradually becomes accustomed to feeds which are too large and, ceasing to vomit them, begins to show signs of overfeeding and indigestion.

GASTRIC IRRITATION

The infantile gastric mucous membrane is sensitive, and occasionally food is rejected when its *temperature* is higher or lower than the child is accustomed to, especially the latter. The *quantity* of food which the stomach can retain at one time varies with different infants. There are some who either have exceptionally small stomachs, or are exceptionally sensitive to distension. These can take a small feed and digest it perfectly well, but consistently vomit when a larger amount is pressed upon them. They must be fed with small amounts at frequent intervals like premature babies. They nearly all become normal later on.

The *quality* of food is the chief determining factor in gastric irritation. Here there is shown a wide field for personal idiosyncrasy. In artificial feeding the innumerable varieties and modifications of milk have their successes and failures which bear no fixed relationship to their theoretical value. Raw milk is consistently vomited by one baby, dry milk by a second, a complex synthetic preparation by a third, though each one has been prepared, diluted, etc., with due regard to theoretical requirements. Yet another baby will take anything it is offered and thrive.

Apart from this personal factor, the cause of vomiting may be in the excess of one particular constituent, e.g. *fat.*

Even in breast-feeding the milk may be too rich, especially if the mother is taking a diet containing a lot of protein. In artificial feeding the coarsely granuled fat of cow's cream is not always tolerated well at first, and is a frequent cause of vomiting and indigestion. It may be necessary to keep the percentage of fat low until toleration has been established.

Curd Indigestion

Curd indigestion has been spoken of in the chapter on Artificial Feeding. An infant when first introduced to the large, tough curd of cow's casein frequently vomits, especially if there has been no modification of the curd by the use of sodium citrate, dextrin, malto-dextrin, starch, or the process of peptonisation.

Excess of *sugar* may cause vomiting. Any *impurities* in the milk may irritate the gastric mucous membrane ; such are bacteria and the products of bacterial decomposition.

Gastritis in young infants may be preliminary to an inflammatory attack on the whole gastro-intestinal tract. In the majority of these cases the symptoms of gastritis are early and violent, but do not last long ; they give place to intestinal symptoms and the vomiting ceases. In others vomiting persists for some time, and the outlook is more unfavourable. The worst cases occur in epidemic form. In children after early infancy gastritis frequently occurs without any apparent involvement of the bowel, and may be most obstinate. It arises most often as the result of errors in diet, but some-times comes on as a complication or sequela of infectious diseases, especially influenza, measles, and whooping cough, and may be the result of swallowing infected sputa. It is evidenced by loss of appetite, epigastric pain, vomiting, furred tongue, sallow complexion, and general peevishness.

CONSTIPATION

Constipation may by itself cause vomiting, though as a rule there is some associated gastritis. But when these two symptoms, i.e. vomiting and constipation, occur together and do not respond readily to treatment an investigation into possible causes, such as hypertrophic pyloric stenosis or meningitis, must be made.

CONGENITAL HYPERTROPHIC PYLORIC STENOSIS

Congenital hypertrophic pyloric stenosis, occur-ring chiefly in male infants, manifests itself towards the end of the first month of life. Vomiting gradually becomes more frequent and more violent, and is at last projectile in character. Constipation inevitably results, and the infant wastes rapidly. If the possibility of this condition is always kept in mind these cases should be diagnosed early, as the peristaltic wave moving from left to right across and down the abdomen is easily seen, and with patience the pyloric tumour may be felt. The earlier the diagnosis is made the better, as surgical treatment is now almost universally adopted (Rammstedt's operation), and should be performed while the child is still in a fit condition.

Pylorospasm, or Achalasia of the Pylorus

Pylorospasm, or achalasia of the pylorus, is a condition which closely simulates hypertrophic stenosis, but is entirely functional. There is no hypertrophy of muscle, and the pyloric spasm, though it may be sustained for some time, relaxes entirely when it does relax. There is generally associated hyperchlorhydria, indeed this may be the cause of the condition. Pylorospasm also occurs a few weeks after birth, and the vomiting may be projectile in character. Either constipation or diarrhœa may be present ; there is no peristalsis, though the shape of the stomach may be seen very definitely after a meal and some indefinite churning movements ; there is no pyloric tumour.

Treatment.—Breast-feeding or a simple easily-digested milk preparation, small doses of sodium bicarbonate before feeds to neutralise the hyper-acidity, together with a minim of tincture of belladonna as an anti-spasmodic. If the child is a boy, it should be circumcised ; this alone sometimes serves to relieve the spasm.

Nervous Vomiting

Nervous vomiting is only diagnosed after all the more common causes have been excluded. It is, of course, quite impossible to prove that there is such a thing as functional vomiting at such an early age, but most authorities agree that there is. It occurs in the nervous child of a nervous parent, and is easily brought on by any disturbance of the normal routine. These babies are sometimes better away from their mothers except when being breast-fed, and it is even occasionally necessary to wean them if vomiting is persistent. The care of a good placid nurse, fresh air, and an undisturbed routine, generally cure the condition. Bromides may be given at first :

R̸ Sod. Bromidi . . . . gr. ij
Aq. ad. . . . . . ʒj

three times a day to a baby of three months old.

Cerebral and Symptomatic Vomiting

Cerebral and symptomatic vomiting will not for long simulate the forms of vomiting due to local trouble. The first is present all through the course of meningitis and other acute cerebral affections of infancy ; the second may occur in the early stages of practically all acute infective diseases of childhood, such as scarlet-fever, influenza, pneumonia. Recognition that vomiting is a common early symptom in most of the acute illnesses of children will save the practitioner from making a too hasty diagnosis.

Vomiting is also an early and sometimes persistent symptom in nephritis.

Vomiting is associated with affections of the peritoneum, especially when the condition is acute. The commonest peritoneal infection in childhood is appendicitis; after that, acute tuberculous and acute pneumococcic infections.

Gastric ulcer is extremely rare, but cases as young as five months have been reported.

CHAPTER IX

PREMATURE INFANTS

PREMATURITY, which is largely responsible for a high infant mortality, is chiefly due to maternal causes.

These may be : Trauma, either physical or mental, prolonged malnutrition, any acute disease, certain chronic diseases, such as tuberculosis, nephritis and especially syphilis, operation for other than pelvic conditions, diabetes, etc., etc. The occurrence of multiple pregnancy and malposition of the fœtus in utero may also be causes of premature labour.

One should distinguish, especially in giving a prognosis, between the infant that is fundamentally healthy, but is born before its time owing to accident, induction, etc., and the infant that has the added handicap either of some definite constitutional disease, such as syphilis, or of continued malnutrition in utero, due to the mother's ill-health.

In the former the various functions are not fully developed and the child is not ready for extra-uterine life ; it takes, therefore, more than the six weeks or so of prematurity to bring it into the normal condition of the full-time baby, but it can, in time and with care, develop into perfect normality and may eventually become as robust as any other child. The latter has a poor chance ; it either dies within a few weeks of birth, or drags out a difficult childhood with a low vitality and a lack of resistance to the traumas of everyday life.

The Premature Infant

Estimation of the age of a premature infant cannot always be satisfactorily based upon the history of the mother, though this together with the events of pregnancy, quickening, etc., must be taken into account. A child becomes viable at about the twenty-eighth week; if born previous to this, it may live for a few minutes, but not more. It is at this time bright red in colour, much wrinkled, and covered with an abundance of lanugo. If born between the twenty-ninth and thirty-second week, the testicles will be found in the scrotum (in males), and ossification of the lower epiphysis of the femur will have begun. The latter point, viz. the ossification of the first epiphysis, makes a fairly definite date in fœtal life and may easily be established by X-rays in cases where it is important to know the fœtal age. Between the thirty-second and thirty-sixth weeks the wrinkles begin to smooth out and the nails reach the tips of the fingers.

Ossification of the skeletal system proceeds in definite order during fœtal life, beginning with the appearance of the first centre in the clavicle at the sixth or seventh week. By the use of X-rays Hess has made a complete study of the order of ossification; his tables, diagrams, and radiograms may be studied in his book, *Premature and Congenitally Diseased Infants*.

The weight and length of premature infants are unreliable data for the estimation of age, but

the head circumference is more constant. Von
Winckel gives the measurements as :

28 weeks old	9 –11 inches
32 ,, ,, ...	10 –12 inches
36 ,, ,, ...	11½–13 inches
40 ,, ,, ...	13 –15 inches

Symptoms.—One of the most noticeable facts
about premature infants is the weakness of their
respiratory efforts. This is partly due to weak
muscular power and partly to the deficient development of the respiratory centres. The result is,
that only part of the lung is used, and it is several
weeks before complete expansion takes place. During
this time apnœic attacks may occur from time to
time. They are of bad omen. The rate of respiration in the premature infant varies between 40
and 50. The heart is relatively well-developed,
though the ductus arteriosus, which should close
during the first forty-eight hours, often remains
open for considerably longer. The pulse rate
averages 120. Sucking and swallowing ability are
low, and the infant soon becomes tired and gives up
the effort. On the other hand, preparation for
digestion is fairly complete, as pepsin, hydrochloric
acid, and rennin are all found in the stomach quite
early in fœtal life. Both thymus and thyroid
glands are fully developed.

The heat-regulating mechanism is deficient in these
babies ; the tendency is for them to lose heat, and
there is some difficulty in keeping the extremities
at a reasonable temperature ; on the other hand,
it is quite easy to raise the temperature too much and

to find a sudden rise to 104° Fahr. or more as a result of too many hot-water bottles and blankets.

There is, unfortunately, a marked tendency to hæmorrhages in these infants, possibly owing to weak vascular walls and diminished coagulability of the blood ; these hæmorrhages predispose to infection.

Pathological Changes.—Apart from specific diseases and congenital abnormalities the most noticeable lesions to be found in the bodies of premature infants are hæmorrhages. These may occur in any of the organs, in the pleura, or scattered through the substance of the lung, in the kidneys, intestines, liver, etc. They are frequently intracranial, and in this situation may be looked upon as a common cause of death. When death does not occur early, the clots may readily become infected and lead to meningitis, brain abscess, etc. Where the issue is not fatal, after results may produce syndromes such as spastic diplegia.

DISEASES OF THE PREMATURE

Respiratory.—A certain amount of atelectasis may be looked upon as normal for the first few weeks of a premature infant's life ; it is evinced by shallow breathing, some falling in of the chest wall during inspiration, and, on auscultation, a poor respiratory murmur with the addition of many crepitant râles ; the percussion note is rarely impaired. Exaggerated or prolonged atelectasis will cause attacks of asphyxia or cyanosis and will probably prove fatal.

Catarrhal infections are readily taken, as the infant seems to have no natural immunity to them.

It cannot be too strongly impressed on the mother that she should take the utmost care to protect the new-born child from contact with people who are suffering from colds, sore throats, and coughs. Broncho-pneumonia is not infrequent in prematures, and is sometimes found post mortem even though no definite signs have been present during life.

Passive congestion of the lung is apt to occur simply from lack of movement ; this is likely to happen if the child is left too long in one position in an incubator. A moderate amount of " picking up " and handling is desirable if it can be carried out in a warm room.

Gastro-intestinal infection is a frequent cause of death, especially in the artificially fed. The organism may be introduced in the milk or by the use of contaminated teats, etc. Stomatitis and thrush are common.

Convulsions may occur shortly after birth. They may be partly functional, but are often due to intracranial hæmorrhages, which are found in a large number of cases. They may be accompanied by various forms of spasmophilia.

Hernia.—Umbilical and inguinal herniæ are commoner in the premature than in the full-time infant.

Mental deficiency in varying grades is found.

Hydrocephalus is sometimes the cause of prematurity. Its origin is uncertain ; it renders parturition difficult, and if progressive leads to marked mental deficiency. It must not be mistaken for megacephalus, which is frequent in premature babies, and only means that at first the head grows at a quicker rate than the body.

Rickets is frequently a complication of prematurity and tends to occur earlier than in full-time children.

Syphilis must always be considered. The clinical picture is often not typical, and it is advisable in all doubtful cases to do a Wassermann reaction on the child's blood.

TREATMENT

The main requirements in the treatment of premature infants are :

1. Warmth, and
2. Human Milk.

If the child is to be treated in hospital the use of the incubator is the safest method, especially in a big ward. Heating the cot by hot-water bottles, electric pads, or electric lights is not so reliable, as it is difficult to keep an even heat, and the child's temperature rises or falls with the surroundings only too readily. We are more concerned here, however, with treatment in the home, and especially in those homes where expensive apparatus cannot be obtained. The mother should be advised to pad her cot well with layers of cotton wool, which may be covered with jaconet. If the cot is not a wide, roomy one it would be better to use an open washing basket or even a large box, as there must be room for three or four hot-water bottles at an ample distance from the child, and well protected by flannel coverings. If the water bottles are refilled in rotation the temperature may be kept reasonably even without much difficulty. All coverings should be wool, warm but light. The child should be wrapped in cotton wool, covered by knitted wool vest, coat, etc., and the napkins should be of flannelette or lint. The head must be kept covered. Bathing in water must be avoided for the first few days (some say the first few weeks), and in place of bathing the body is oiled over every day. While it is important so to arrange the clothing that it may be easily and quickly changed in order to prevent unnecessary manipulation, it is unwise to leave the child lying in one position in its cot for too long. From time to time it must be turned over, and when the room is quite warm and free from draughts it should be picked up and carried about.

FEEDING

There is generally some difficulty in establishing breast-feeding where premature birth has occurred, and even more in sustaining it. As the flow of milk can only be kept up by emptying the breast regularly, and as the feeble infant cannot do this itself, pumping or expression will probably have to be used for some time. The premature infant should be fed every 2 or 2½ hours during the day and may often have to be wakened for the feed. Where practicable the child should be weighed before feeding, put to the breast, and when it has sucked as much as its strength will allow weighed again. The breast should then be emptied either by pump or by expression, and the feed, if it has been too small, may now be made up to the desired amount by giving part of the remaining breast milk with a small bottle or pipette. The other breast is emptied in the same way at the next feed. With care and patience during the first few weeks a regular flow may be kept up until the infant is strong enough to take a complete feed by itself.

Unfortunately the child is frequently only brought to the Welfare Centre after the breast milk has failed and the mother has already started on the difficult path of artificial feeding. The problems of artificial feeding for the premature are much the same as for normal infants, and are referred to in the chapter on that subject.

CHAPTER X

RICKETS

ETIOLOGY

DURING the last few years a considerable amount of research work has been done on rickets and many interesting and useful facts have been established, especially with regard to the effect of various treatments. The etiology, however, remains obscure; we call it a deficiency disease, but it is not yet at all clear what is deficient, nor can the pathological processes be adequately explained.

Very little is seen of rickets before the fifth month of life; the usual age of onset is between eight and eighteen months. It occurs early, however, in premature babies, in babies suffering from congenital syphilis, and in all those who have suffered from any acute illness during the early months, e.g. broncho-pneumonia, whooping cough, measles.

There is a certain *familial* tendency; true the same surroundings and same methods of up-bringing might account for some cases where every child of a family gets rickets, but it cannot explain all cases, especially as a careful mother who has had one baby with rickets is generally eager to avoid it with the others.

FEEDING

Breast-fed babies are least affected, but they are by no means immune. In the poorest classes

where breast-feeding is an economy it is carried on
for a year or eighteen months, but there is nothing
to take its place when the child is weaned, fresh
milk is rarely seen, and the diet after the first year
chiefly consists of bread, margarine, and tea with
a dash of condensed skimmed milk.   The rickets of
breast-fed babies, therefore, develops at a late age,
and is not generally the severest kind.

With artificial feeding rickets is very commonly
associated.   Many attempts have been made to
discover whether a deficiency or an excess of any
particular food element can be regarded as a causative
factor.   Formerly it was considered that deficiency
of fat in the food was a common cause of rickets ;
deficiency of proteins was also suggested ; and excess
of carbohydrate was yet another possible fault.
Latterly the deficiency has been thought to be
rather one of vitamine content, especially the so-
called anti-rachitic Vitamine A.   Young animals fed
on a diet which is wholly deficient in vitamines
rarely fail to develop rickets within a short period.
Necessarily the only systematic and truly scientific
experiments that can be carried out with controls
are those upon animals ; abundant work has been
done with feeding experiments on puppies and rats.
Helpful though this work has been, it would be a
mistake to imagine that the feeding of babies could
be entirely based upon the requirements of young
puppies, etc.

Practical experience shows that the worst cases of
rickets occur in children who have been reared on
sweetened condensed milk and on patent malted
wheat foods ; the latter have often been given with
much diluted milk or even with water only.   There

are, however, plenty of cases occurring after raw milk or dried milk feeding, even when there have been careful supervision and regulation.

It seems probable that *over-feeding* is sometimes a causal factor. Rickets is by no means confined to the poorer classes ; many well-to-do babies get attacked, though the disease is not generally allowed to develop so far. There are plenty of folk who think you cannot have too much of a good thing, and it is possible that rickets is induced by the large quantities of milk forced upon fat babies in homes where money is no object. Mothers and nurses do not seem to realise that when a child is embarking on a mixed diet towards the end of its first year there is no necessity to continue giving the same amount of milk as it had before. One often meets with babies who are still taking a quart of milk a day in spite of the fact that they are also getting two solid meals in the shape of rusks, egg, fruit, gravies, etc.

LACK OF FRESH AIR AND SUNLIGHT

Lack of fresh air and sunlight are potent factors in the production of rickets.

Rickets is known to occur principally during the winter and spring ; new cases are rarely seen during the summer. More than that, if the summer has been unusually wet and sunless there is a marked increase of cases and an earlier incidence during the following winter. If a close inquiry be made into the circumstances of rickets cases many instances will be found of : (1) basement rooms ; (2) tenement dwellings with no yard or garden ; (3) overworked mothers unable to take the baby out for more than half an hour a day ; or (4) in the case of well-to-do people, a hot stuffy nursery and outings in a deep-hooded pram on fine days only.

Over-clothing

Over-clothing may be considered a probable contributory cause, inasmuch as it leads to over-heating, prevention of free skin function, and, in the case of tight clothes, diminished oxygenation by compression of the chest. The garment called " stays," which every child of the poor classes wears from earliest infancy, is a thick quilted affair tightly roped round the thorax and calculated effectually to prevent complete expansion of the lungs.

An important point which has not, perhaps, received sufficient attention is the association of rickets with all acute debilitating diseases of early infancy and even more with congenital disease such as syphilis. A child who has suffered from acute broncho-pneumonia at the age of three or four months may subsequently be treated with the greatest care as to diet, clothing, fresh air, yet after some months begins to show signs of rickets. Early measles, whooping cough, gastro-enteritis are all frequently followed by rickets, while in cases of congenital syphilis it is almost impossible to avoid some tendency towards the disease during the first year of life. It would seem that anything which tends to lower general resistance (including prematurity) lays the child open to this fault of metabolism.

ENDOCRINE GLANDS

The association of tetany with rickets suggests the possibility of some fault of the parathyroid glands, especially in view of their known influence on calcium metabolism.

However this may be in theory, the exhibition of parathyroid gland extract does not seem to do anything towards curing the condition.

MANIFESTATIONS

There are not a few cases in which rickets affects mainly the osseous system, and leads to very little disturbance of the general health. These are generally comparatively late in onset, beginning between a year and eighteen months. The child is fat and well-coloured; a certain amount of atonia of the muscles occurs, but he continues to get about quite happily, rapidly developing bowing of the legs. The epiphyses are enlarged, but the skull changes are not quite so noticeable at this age, and the teeth that have already erupted do not decay.

These children become remarkably bow-legged and are often not brought up for treatment until late. They respond well to light and cod-liver oil, and straighten out to an extent that would have been thought impossible at first sight of the case.

Mainly, however, rickets causes a general disturbance of metabolism in which almost every part of the body suffers. Its development may be noticed in the early stages by the watchful medical officer and diagnosed before any gross bony changes occur.

8

General Symptoms

The child is fretful and peevish during the day, restless at night. *Sweating* is an early sign, chiefly noticed during sleep, and especially on the head. There is often no wasting of the sub-cutaneous fat, but the muscles waste considerably, and become *atonic* to such a degree that movements and positions already accomplished are abandoned, e.g. the baby of eight months ceases to sit up, the boy of a year old " goes off his legs."

Anæmia is variable ; it is usually present in some degree, and may be so marked as to suggest Splenic Anæmia Infantum, though the blood picture is somewhat different. There is occasionally a general enlargement of the *sub-cutaneous glands*.

Gastro-intestinal manifestations are common, probably due to a general lack of resistance to catarrhal organisms. Thus, the baby may suffer from chronic or sub-acute diarrhœa, vomiting, colic. The liver and spleen are generally enlarged to some extent, but a marked enlargement of the spleen is not a usual feature. The " pot-belly " is mainly due to slackness of the muscles of the abdominal wall, but also partly to flatulence and loss of intestinal tone, partly to the large liver.

Catarrhs of the Respiratory Tract are also frequent, naso-pharynx, larynx, trachea, and bronchi all taking part. Bronchitis may become a chronic condition in the rickety child, and is particularly vicious in that it combines with the softening of the ribs and falling-in of the thorax to produce partial collapse of the lungs and deficient air entry. More acute attacks upon the lung may result in broncho-pneumonia, one of the most dreaded complications of rickets and perhaps the most frequent cause of death.

Nervous manifestations are :—

1. *Tetany*.—This is a term applied to a curious contraction of the muscles of hands and feet. The hand is flexed, the fingers extended, while the small muscles of the thumb pull it closely across the palm of the hand. The foot is also hyper-extended, the toes flexed. The muscles affected are in constant condition of hyper-tonus and only relax during deep sleep

2. *Laryngismus stridulus*.—This is a nervous contraction of laryngeal muscles which for the time being inhibits inspiration entirely. It comes on suddenly, unassociated with cough or the swallowing of food, etc. The spasm lasts several seconds while cyanosis rapidly increases, then relaxes as suddenly, when a deep inspiration is taken and the child is quickly relieved. It is a condition which is probably allied to asthma, but it is most often met with in children suffering from rickets.

3. *Convulsions*.—The unbalanced nervous system of these babies makes them peculiarly liable to convulsions, though there is generally some more immediate determining cause, such as indiscretions of diet.

4. *Facial Irritability*.—This is a sign, not a symptom. Tapping on the main trunk of the facial nerve, just in front of the ear, produces contraction of all the muscles on that side of the face. It is merely an evidence of increased irritability of the nerve.

Osseous System

Here the changes are the most obvious though, perhaps, the least disturbing to the general well-being of the child. They are important, clinically, as they serve as good indicators of the progress or healing of the disease. The epiphyses of the long bones are all enlarged, including those of the ribs (rickety rosary) ; this is due to an excessive growth activity, with, however, deficient ossification.

The shafts are soft and have a tendency to bend in the direction determined by the weight of the body and by the action of the stronger groups of muscles.

The thorax becomes deformed as a whole. There is frequently lateral flattening producing an artificial prominence of the sternum, while a transverse depression occurs just above the level of the liver, known as Harrison's sulcus. This general retraction of the chest wall is partly caused and certainly kept up by the frequent bronchial catarrh which makes efficient expansion of the lungs impossible.

The pelvis becomes flattened at this time, though the effects are not noticeable until adult life.

The flat bones of the skull are subject to the same rapid formation of imperfect bone tissue, but only in their centres ; growth at the edges is considerably retarded. The result is a skull with bosses in the frontal and parietal regions, and a widely open anterior fontanelle.

The eruption of the teeth is sometimes delayed, though in many cases the incisors, at least, are already cut before the onset of the disease. What is more disastrous is that the teeth are of a poor quality and decay early.

The X-ray appearances should be studied carefully ; they are most valuable indications of the severity of the disease and of the progress in treatment.

Unfortunately only a few well-equipped Welfare Centres have the advantage of possessing the apparatus, but it should be possible to arrange for one X-ray plant to be shared by a group of centres, or failing that, arrangements should be made to obtain facilities from the nearest hospital. While the disease is active the epiphyseal line in the long bones is seen to be blurred and softened, the shaft is rarefied, the compact bone thinned ; the extent of the bowing may be clearly seen. When healing is taking place the epiphyseal line gradually resumes its sharp outline, while the process of buttressing the bone by sub-periosteal growth on the concave surfaces can be watched.

TREATMENT

Given the co-operation of the parents treatment is very hopeful. It is now generally accepted that the two most effective weapons are cod-liver oil and ultra-violet rays. A good brand of cod-liver oil should be chosen, and may be given combined with malt, or as a simple emulsion (50%), or combined with iron or with compound hypophosphites. Most children will take one or other of these forms, but a few are found who invariably reject cod-liver oil. These should be given a glycerine extract of the vitamins of cod-liver oil, which has recently been put on the market under the name of Ostelin.

Ultra-violet rays may be given by a mercury

vapour lamp or by a carbon arc lamp. Exposure should be made three times a week, care being taken to begin with small doses until the child's tolerance is known.

The results are so uniformly good that the treatment may be looked upon as essential (always supposing that direct sun-light cannot be obtained), and no Welfare Centre can be complete without this apparatus, which may be used beneficially, not only for rickets, but for all cases of malnutrition, chronic septic conditions, tuberculosis, etc.

Meanwhile the institution of special light treatment must not excuse the Medical Officer from giving detailed instructions as to the general care of the child. He must not rest content until he has made the mother realise that she is to give the infant as much fresh air and light as she can possibly manage. The visiting nurse will pursue the same subject whenever she makes a call. Clothing must be supervised, all tight garments and all unnecessary garments abandoned. Diet must be carefully planned to include reasonable proportions of all the food elements. Exercise of the limbs should be encouraged. Here arises a difficulty; it is undesirable to allow a child to put its weight on to the softened and bending leg bones. Yet it is impossible to prevent a year-old baby from getting on to its feet whenever it is left free to do so, except in the early stages when all desire for walking is absent. The use of splints is advocated and they seem to be necessary for the first few weeks if a child insists on standing without them. It is important that during this time massage and passive movement should be carried out regularly, to take the place of natural movements. As soon as the healing process of the bone condition is established, even though bowing is still present (here the X-ray picture is a definite help), the splints should be discontinued and the muscles used freely. I would rather see splints left off too soon than too late.

Massage is a most useful part of the treatment and may be used throughout.

CHAPTER XI

RASHES IN INFANCY

FROM the earliest days of life the delicate skin of the infant is most susceptible to internal and external influences. It reacts quickly to modifications of temperature, irritation, microbic and toxic invasions. It becomes, therefore, one of the common duties of the clinic medical officer to examine and diagnose a multitudinous variety of rashes which may frequently puzzle him even after years of experience. The following are a few of the more common skin conditions found at an early age.

"GUM RASH"

This popular term is loosely used for a number of different conditions and often for lichen urticatus. It is most often applied to a rash which has as yet earned no title for itself in the books on dermatology, partly because it is rarely treated seriously by mothers, who regard it as one of the inevitable complaints of infancy. It takes the form of groups of small red papules, sometimes with an erythematous background, which appear on the exposed parts, chiefly on the face. They occur very early, in the first few weeks, and are apparently not irritating, as far as one can judge in such young infants. I associate them entirely with dirt, as they are not seen in well-cared-for babies, and examination will

nearly always reveal filthy black finger-nails, dirt
in the crevices of the hands, and musty garments.
The infection is probably staphylococcal, and this
is the first protest of the skin against a heavy invasion.
Sometimes the papules become pustular.

Sweat Rash

Sweat Rash is common enough, especially in the
summer. The distribution is chiefly in the folds
of the skin, the axillæ, groins, neck. There is a
moist erythematous surface, with scattered papules
or vesicles which afterwards dry up and desquamate.
It generally indicates that the clothes have been too
thick or have been made of unsuitable material,
which does not allow ready evaporation of sweat.
The rash is best treated with a mild non-irritating
powder, and readjustment of the clothing.

Irritative Dermatitis

This may be produced by strong alkaline soaps,
or by harsh woollen clothes, or as a result of washing
the under garments in soda. These details should
all be inquired into when papulo-erythematous
rashes occur which cannot be accounted for in any
other way. They are not always easy to dissociate
from sweat rashes, but are more diffuse and may
occur all over the body and limbs. In this group
one might include the irritative erythema which
often occurs as the result of rubbing strong camphorated oil on the chest. When a baby gets a
cold its mother's first idea is to " soak it in camphorated oil," as she herself expresses it. The rash,
which is often induced thereby, is, of course, limited
to chest, back, and part of the abdomen. If mothers

must use camphorated oil they should be instructed to dilute it with the same quantity of olive oil.

Eczema

Infantile eczema is not present at birth, but develops early as a rule, though some cases are delayed until the eighth or ninth month. It has much the same characters as the eczema of adults, but a different distribution. There is first an intense erythema, followed by multiple fissuring of the epidermis and oozing of serum which subsequently dries into crusts. Sometimes groups of papules form, which go through the respective phases of vesicle and pustule and dry up, leaving large scabs. The variation between " dry " and " moist " eczema is merely one of degree, the dry cases being those in which the serous oozing is not a marked feature. There is intense itching, and the lesion, primarily non-bacterial, can readily become infected. In babies the rash is chiefly over the head and face, encroaching a little on the neck ; only in very severe cases does it spread over the body. On the face it often gives a mask-like appearance as it does not affect the eyelids, lips, or nostrils. In infancy it is not difficult to diagnose as the only other abnormal condition of the scalp likely to occur so early is a diffuse, scurfy condition, in which greenish-yellow, greasy masses collect round the roots of the hair, chiefly over the fontanelle. This is not inflammatory, and is non-irritable. Later in childhood, eczema might well be confused with an extensive chronic impetigo which sometimes spreads over the whole scalp.

Most cases of infantile eczema yield to treatment ;

they recur two or three times, but generally clear up altogether after the first year. Some cases continue into later childhood, and the subject is liable to develop asthma later in life.

The treatment is an expectant one. Keep the surface protected, especially from scratching and rubbing, do not allow it to be washed with water, and cover with a thick layer of some mild ointment, Ung. Petrolei Co., or a zinc oxide ointment made up with plenty of starch. Attend to the diet, as it is possible that therein lies the cause of the complaint. Very small doses (gr. $\frac{1}{3}$ to gr. $\frac{1}{8}$ daily) of thyroid extract have been found beneficial.

LICHEN URTICATUS (STROPHULUS, NETTLE-RASH)

This is one of the commonest and at the same time the most mysterious of children's rashes. It occurs in successive crops of papules chiefly on the trunk (the buttocks commonly), but is also seen on the limbs and much more rarely on the face. The papules, which are large, are at first surrounded by a vivid ring of erythema, and in bad cases are surmounted by a bleb filled with serum. They are intensely irritable. The crop, consisting of from five to fifteen separate papules, is acutely inflamed for about twenty-four hours, then gradually fades; but the raised spots, though ceasing to be irritable, can be felt in the skin for over a week. Other crops succeed, and the child may be troubled with them for several weeks at a time. When scratched and broken they may become very septic. They interfere with the child's rest owing to their extreme irritability. Children may have this rash as early as the third or fourth month, and will be liable to recurring attacks for three or four years; they are rarely seen after the sixth year. There is a marked seasonal incidence; the first warm weather, generally in May, brings large numbers of babies to the Welfare Centre with this complaint, and it continues through the summer months until September. Only occasionally does an especially susceptible child suffer from lichen urticatus throughout the winter.

The cause has not yet been discovered. Perfectly healthy breast-fed babies suffer as well as those artificially fed. Gastro-intestinal disturbance has been regarded as a probable cause, but it will be found that the majority have perfectly normal stools, though there are bound to be some among such numbers with an irregularity, in the form of constipation, offensive stools, etc. The general health does not seem to suffer, except from lack of sleep. Certainly no treatment for the bowel has been found of any permanent use.

It seems likely that lichen urticatus may be allied to other urticarial lesions and may be an expression of intolerance on the part of the child to some one element of its food.

Attempts at tracking the particular susceptibility have, however, not been very successful up to the present. The fact that children all grow out of it in a few years lends colour to the view, as it may be assumed that toleration is gradually established.

Treatment.—The bath should be given in the morning instead of night, as warm water increases the irritation; the spots may be dabbed from time to time with calamine lotion. Any bowel defect that may be present should be treated. Gastro-intestinal anti-septics such as guaiacol, salol, kerol, dimol, and small doses of mercurial compounds have been given, but, in the author's hands, have had no effect. With children on a mixed diet some attempt should be made to trace possible causes in the diet which preceded the onset.

SCABIES

Scabies may attack children of all ages, and is similar to lichen urticatus in being intensely irritable, especially at night. In its early stages typical burrows can often be seen, but a child's skin reacts very vigorously to the invasion, and often a mass of small pustules and dried scabs obliterate the original signs. The rash should be especially looked for between the fingers and in the folds of the wrist. In young infants the infection spreads rapidly over the whole body, and even the face is attacked. The best confirmation of a scabies diagnosis is the history of similar irritating spots in other members of the family.

This is a difficult condition to deal with in infants, as the drugs necessary to kill the acarus are liable to cause dermatitis in a delicate skin. If sulphur is used, the ointment should not be applied for more than two nights in succession, and then there should be several days interval before another application.

One sees a lot of sulphur dermatitis due to indiscriminate treatment of scabies.

IMPETIGO

Impetigo need only be mentioned briefly. It is not very likely to be mistaken for any other rash, except in the case, already mentioned, of a chronic impetiginous scalp simulating eczema. The ordinary variety appears at the mouth, nose, ears, scalp, etc., and is generally characteristic.

In its treatment the main point seems to be to prevent the child from touching the spots. The arms may be splinted for the purpose.

Napkin Rashes

These may be caused by :

1. Irritating urine.
2. Hyper-acid stools.
3. Alkaline stools.

1. In cases of " scalding urine," the rash is found all over the area covered by the napkin, and frequently on the calves and heels as well, since these parts are drawn up against the wet napkin. The skin is bright red and rather shiny in appearance ; if neglected it may go on to superficial ulceration. The folds of skin are protected, so generally escape ; this is an important point in the diagnosis from congenital syphilis or from seborrhœic dermatitis.

In a boy a red, sore prepuce helps to indicate the source of the trouble.

2. Acidity of the stool is produced by excessive fermentation ; it leads to a bright erythema round the anus and over any part of the skin with which the stool comes into contact. Excoriation takes place rapidly, and there is soon a widely spread weeping surface of superficial ulceration.

3. The alkaline stool, which is evidence of protein dyspepsia, produces rather a different picture. There is less erythema but more ulceration, the

ulcers appearing in groups, round, punched-out, and rather deep.

Treatment.—The diet must be adjusted according to the kind of stool being passed. Napkins must be changed frequently. A mild ointment should be applied, e.g. :

R/	Ol. Ricini	.	.	.	.	.	℥ij
	Ung. Zinci	.	.	.	.	.	℥j
	Ung. Acidi Borici	.	.	.	.	℥j

About 20 minims of Tinct. Benz. Co. may be added to this if ulcers are slow to heal.

SYPHILIS

A bullous syphilide may appear a few days after birth and is usually fatal, but the commoner rash is one that does not show itself until about the third week—sometimes later still, but not later than the third month. It is similar to that of acquired syphilis, beginning as erythematous patches, which later become raised and slightly scaly ; they vary in colour from pink to copper. They may become markedly impetiginous. The distribution is important ; beginning over the buttocks and perineum, the patches may at first simulate a napkin erythema, but in the case of syphilis there is as much, if not more, rash in the folds than on the convex surfaces.

The face is attacked early and the mouth shows mucous patches and radiating fissures which have a typical appearance. The soles and palms are almost invariably involved, showing discoloured patches, from which the skin peels in thick flakes. Muco-purulent rhinitis is invariably present, and occasion-ally enlarged glands may be felt.

Seborrhœic Dermatitis

Seborrhœic dermatitis, though not common in babies, does occasionally occur on the napkin area, giving rise to rather greasy-looking patches, chiefly in the folds of skin. If this is suspected, examine the mother, as she is probably suffering from seborrhœa of the scalp.

The Exanthemata

The Exanthemata need not be described in detail here. Every medical man when faced with a rash will cast his mind over the possibility of measles, rubella, scarlet-fever, etc. In all cases it is safer to take the temperature and examine the throat. The history of contact, the onset, the general appearance, and distribution of the rash must all be taken into account.

CHAPTER XII

THERE are few more embarrassing situations for the medical practitioner than to be confronted with a case of pyrexia in a young child, with no other obvious symptoms or signs. Children are notably more unstable with regard to their body temperature than adults, and are apt to show a reaction which seems altogether out of proportion to the cause.

Each case has to be considered as possibly a serious one, and investigated not only very thoroughly but with the least possible delay, in view of the fact that in certain conditions, e.g. cerebro-spinal meningitis, an early diagnosis may make all the difference between a fatal and a favourable termination.

TEETHING

Whereas the layman has seized upon teething as the *fons et origo* of nearly all infantile ailments and complaints, the medical man has rather gone to the opposite extreme and declares that teething, being a natural physiological process, is unassociated with pathological symptoms, and that any bodily ills which may occur during dentition have no actual connection with that process.

The first conception is of course absurd. From about the age of five months to two or two and a

9   129

half years all children are teething ; the process is more or less continuous, and as soon as one tooth is through another is beginning to thrust forward. Teething is, therefore, a plausible excuse for almost any complaint during this period. On the other hand, although many children seem to cut their teeth with little or no discomfort, it can hardly be denied that in others the process produces a remarkable amount of pain and malaise. A child who is normal in other respects will have a few days of general irritability, loss of appetite, copious dribbling, and constant thumb-biting. The symptoms then subside, a small sharp point can be felt in the gum, and the rest of the tooth proceeds to push through without further trouble. These attacks often occur two or three times before the tooth makes an appearance. The temperature is frequently raised—sometimes to 101° or more. During painful dentition the child is apt to stuff the fingers into the ears or to pull the lobes, and to roll the head from side to side, thus leading the parents to suppose that there is some trouble with the ears or brain.

DIGESTIVE DISTURBANCES

The temperature balance is much upset by the ingestion of food which either in quality or quantity is unsuitable to the child's digestive mechanism, and probably one of the commonest causes of short, febrile attacks is an error in diet. This is all the more likely to occur if the child's stomach has not done what it usually has the good sense to do—viz. vomited all of its contents to get rid of the offending material. In these cases the sooner the bowel is emptied the better, and, happily, the giving of a purge is, with few exceptions, a safe method of treatment in the early stage of fever, so that even if the diagnosis is not correct no harm has been done. These disturbances are probably due to an excess of one of the food elements or to unsuitability of a particular food.

Ptomaine Poisoning, which may also cause an acute rise of temperature, comes under another category. In this condition there is a virulent chemical toxin or bactero-toxin which, quickly absorbed, leads to a profound general disturbance as well as a local reaction. *Infective gastro-enteritis*, occurring chiefly in the weeks between mid-July and the end of September, generally starts with a rise of temperature; it is not as a rule difficult to diagnose, though it must be remembered that many infective diseases start with diarrhœa or vomiting. *Constipation* alone may give rise to slight pyrexia, but not when it is a chronic condition.

MENINGITIS

The onset of cerebro-spinal meningitis may be very insidious in the young child. There is usually pyrexia, but the symptoms are only of a vague, general character at first, vomiting, constipation, fretfulness, and general malaise. When definite head retraction, rigidity, strabismus, etc., have set in the diagnosis is not difficult, but it is important to come to a conclusion before this, and points to be specially noticed are the bulging fontanelle (in infants) and the staring look of the eyes, both early signs. In all doubtful cases it is well to do a lumbar puncture and have the fluid examined for globulin, cells, chlorides, sugar, and bacteria. In the case of cerebro-spinal meningitis the earlier the diagnosis is established the better, as treatment by withdrawal of fluid and injection of the specific antitoxic serum has very considerably lowered the death rate in this disease, even in quite young infants.

Otitis Media

In a child who is old enough to complain and to indicate the locality of his pain the ear-ache of otitis media does not often pass unnoticed, but in the infant no such help is given, and it should be one of the rules of the medical practitioner never to omit the examination of the ears in a febrile infant where the cause of the pyrexia is not apparent. The external auditory meatus is short and the tympanum can be easily seen with a good reflected light, though sometimes a small speculum is necessary. The bright red, bulging membrane is evidence of acute inflammation, probably originating in the naso-pharynx, and the tension may easily be relieved by puncture under an anæsthetic. It is true that in the majority of cases the membrane will burst in any case, thereby relieving the symptoms and discharging the pus, but there is always a danger that this will not occur and that, instead, the infection will track inwards, causing mastoiditis, or meningitis, or cerebral abscess.

Urinary Infections

Infection of the urinary tract is a fairly common event in young infants and frequently goes undiagnosed for a long period, as the symptoms are often obscure. No infant is too young for urinary infection. The offending organism is generally the bacillus coli. Girls are more frequently infected than boys, a fact which suggests that the channel of infection is by the short urethra. In mild cases, where *bacilluria* only is present, there is seldom any rise of temperature, so that this condition need not be considered here. There may, however, be some pyrexia in *b. coli cystitis*, with frequency and pain on micturition. In older children these symptoms are noticeable and early complained of, but in infants they are not so easily detected. A specimen may easily be obtained for examination. It is not necessary to pass a catheter if the urine can be examined within a reasonable period of time after it is passed. The vulva should be clean, and the infant may be held out over a sterilised bowl just after a feed.

By far the most severe infection of the urinary tract is *acute pyelitis*, also caused by the bacillus coli. This may be secondary to cystitis, or may be an acute primary infection. In the latter case the constitutional disturbances are very grave indeed, the high temperature, rigors, vomiting, etc., often completely masking the local symptoms. Perhaps this condition is most often mistaken for appendicitis, but may indeed simulate any highly infective condition, though a rigor is particularly suggestive of pyelitis in children, especially in a country where malaria does not occur.

RHEUMATISM

Since arthritis is not a prominent or a constant feature in the rheumatic attacks of childhood, it is not unusual to find a first attack of rheumatism

difficult to diagnose, the pyrexia being the only
definite sign. In suspected cases care must be taken
to search for nodules, the throat must be examined
for enlarged and unhealthy-looking tonsils, and
salicylates may be given; a rapid improvement
after a sufficiently big dose may help to confirm
the diagnosis.

Once the virus of rheumatism has entered the body
it is not easily thrown out, and, apart from an acute
attack with joint involvement, a child who has once
had rheumatism is very likely to get pyrexial attacks
from time to time, indicating either the retention
of the organism within the tissues, or an increased
susceptibility to re-infection.

TUBERCULOSIS

Tuberculosis in young children offers another
example of " pyrexia of obscure origin." The
disease is usually located in the thoracic glands, and
while the lung is untouched, the symptoms are
vague and indefinite, wasting, anæmia, slight
pyrexia, sweating, sometimes a cough. The physical
signs are even more indefinite, and it is often
impossible to make a diagnosis until the case has
been carefully watched for some time.

In the early stages of *acute pneumonia* it may be
difficult for even the most expert to detect any
abnormal physical signs in the lungs, and the pulse-
respiration ratio is not altered so consistently in
children as in adults. Look out for working of the
alæ nasi, herpes, diminution of urinary chlorides.

The *Exanthemata* may offer difficulties in the
early stages, which are, however, soon solved by
the appearance of their respective rashes. *Influenza*

may be diagnosed during an epidemic, but otherwise should be left till all else fails.

There still remains a number of cases of pyrexia which are not explained by any of the foregoing conditions. Many children have short attacks of feverishness, lasting from a few hours to a few days, with the usual concomitants of fever, viz. headache, lassitude or irritability, loss of appetite, thirst. The mother of six gives a dose of castor oil or a grey powder, and leaves it at that. The more anxious mother calls in the doctor, who, confronted with a temperature of 101°, and not a single physical sign to help him, feels himself to be in an awkward position. He either calls it " a touch of influenza," that convenient refuge for the ignorant, or if he dare to risk his reputation, admits that he does not know. In a few days the temperature has subsided and the child is well again ; the fever is never fully explained. So common are these little febrile attacks among children that they have actually earned a name for themselves in medical textbooks, and may be found described under the heading : " Febricula."

Surely the explanation of this condition is not far to seek. We learn from pathology that the human body is constantly being invaded by pathogenic organisms, that, apart from a certain amount of natural or racial immunity, there is no force wherewith to meet the invaders until the body tissues have been stimulated to produce an antitoxin. If the invading forces are numerous and virulent, some definite illness results, which may or may not be mastered by the resistance of the body in time. If the invading forces are small and the dose of toxin a mild one, there may be no reaction that can be measured in terms of symptoms and signs. But how often must it occur that the body is attacked by unknown organisms, in sufficient strength to give rise to general constitutional distress, rise of temperature, etc., yet unable to make a foothold or to settle down in any organ long enough to produce a definite lesion. In the course of a few days the body conquers, and no sign of the invasion is left, but the individual is the richer for yet another supply of those antitoxins which are to be his chief defence in a germ-ridden world.

CHAPTER XIII

INFANT MORTALITY

THE rate of Infant Mortality in this country is an instructive study for all those who take an interest in Child Welfare. The total rate, the comparative rates in different areas, the causes of death, etc., may be found in detail in the Annual Report of the Registrar General.

It should be remembered that in this connection the word " infant " applies only to children under a year old. The infant mortality rate is the number of infants dying under one year of age, per 1,000 of infants born.

The first point to notice is the steady decrease of mortality from all causes during the last thirty years or more. During the years 1891–1900 the annual rates were between 150 and 160 ; they dropped steadily until in 1913 the rate was 108 per 1,000. The next ten years showed the following figures :—

1914	1915	1916	1917	1918	1919	1920	1921	1922	1923
104	109	91	96	97	89	79	82	77	69

An examination of the rate in various parts of the country gives the following figures during the year 1923 :—

All areas	69
North	85
Middlesex . . .	63
South	55
Wales	74

Analysed still further it is found that the highest rate is in the Northern County Boroughs, 90 for the year, while the lowest is 48 in the South Urban Districts. London in this year gave the figure 61.

The high rates in the Northern and Welsh areas may be accounted for by the conditions of living in thickly populated mining areas. London is remarkably low considering the bad housing conditions, but there is still much to be done to effect a further reduction.

The causes of death are divided into five general classes, while a further analysis is made of the various diseases certified. The five classes, with their mortality rate, are as follow :—

	1914	1915	1916	1917	1918	1919	1920	1921	1922	1923
I. Common Infectious diseases .	6·9	9·0	5·2	5·7	7·9	2·7	4·2	3·6	5·2	4·2
II. Tuberculosis	2·8	2·8	2·3	2·7	1·9	1·6	1·4	1·5	1·3	1·3
III. Diarrhœal diseases .	17·4	15·4	10·5	10·3	9·5	8·7	7·9	13·7	5·5	6·8
IV. Developmental and Wasting diseases .	37·7	37·2	35·6	36·5	35·4	37·4	32·4	33·0	31·4	29·7
V. The rest .	—	—	—	—	—	—	—	—	—	—

The decline in Class I (infectious diseases) is not a very steady one, and the chart, perhaps, covers too short a period for one to be able to judge whether it is a real one. Tuberculosis, never at any time a common condition in the first year of life, shows a slow but gratifyingly steady drop. Diarrhœal

diseases decline rapidly, though in the hot summer
of 1921 there was an abrupt rise to 13·7. This
figure, however, compares very favourably with that

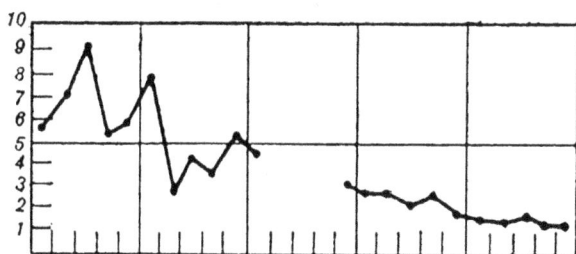

I
INFECTIOUS DISEASES
1913–1923

II
TUBERCULOSIS
1913–1923

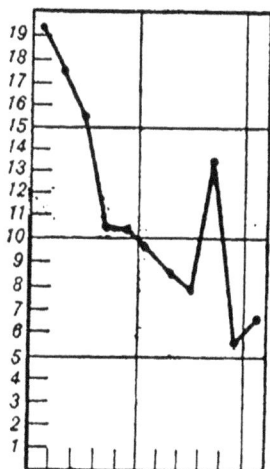

III
DIARRHŒAL DISEASES
1913–1923

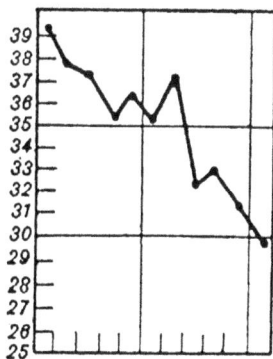

IV
DEVELOPMENTAL AND
WASTING DISEASES
1913–1923

of the summer of 1911, an equally hot, dry summer,
which was as high as 20·0.

The fourth class includes prematurity, and we
may, perhaps, look on the marked decline in this

class during the last four years, as partly due to a decrease in syphilis, which is one of the commonest causes of premature birth.

Deaths from pneumonia, apart from infectious disease, are still high, and do not show any tendency to decline.

Cases labelled " congenital debility " are, however, many fewer than in 1913 ; the numbers have fallen steadily from 12·0 to 9·7. This suggests improved ante-natal care.

Another factor to reckon with is the number of illegitimate births, as the death rate among illegitimate children is always high. In 1923 there were 758,131 total births, and of these 31,522 were illegitimate.

The highest mortality is during the first six months of life ; after that, expectation of life increases slowly but surely.

Neo-natal deaths, i.e. those occurring within one month of birth, are still very numerous—between 20 and 30 per 1,000. After the first year, death rate which is still high is largely attributed to infectious diseases.

In considering these figures one must allow for a good deal of inaccuracy in the certification of cause of disease. Except in hospitals where post-mortem examinations are frequently made to confirm the diagnosis, doctors have little opportunity of assuring themselves that the suspected is the actual cause of death. In children the common causes of death such as pneumonia or gastro-enteritis are generally all too obvious, but there are many acute febrile attacks which end fatally without giving any definite localising symptoms. These get labelled " in-

fluenza," " congestion of the lungs," etc., though
the cause of death is really quite unknown. Wasting
conditions, on the other hand, are probably often
set down as " tuberculosis " without sufficient
proof of the existence of this disease.

Nevertheless the probability is that, in the mass,
the figures are fairly accurate and afford a good
analysis of the infant mortality of this country.

The cause of the decline of the infant death rate
is a question which has been much disputed.
Promoters of Welfare Work naturally point out that
the decline has been most noticeable since the
Notification of Births Act (1907), which marks the
beginning of organised Infant Welfare Work in this
country.   Not only has the work been taken up with
the greatest enthusiasm and thoroughness by local
authorities all over the British Isles, but, what is
more remarkable, it has been met with equal
enthusiasm by the mothers of the country.   The
doubt whether the average working-woman would
ever attend the centres for advice about her children
has been set at rest.   They attend in their thousands,
and their willingness to learn is a revelation.

On the other hand, we must admit that this is
not the sole cause.   Some of the European countries
which have made no special movement in Child
Welfare share with us a present decline in infant
death rate, though possibly not such a rapid one; and
it seems likely that a general preservation of infant
life is the result of an entirely different attitude
taken towards the child, compared with that of
fifty years ago.   The general improvement in the
standard of living might also be taken into account.
Meanwhile there is plenty of work to be done and

many problems to settle, notably that of housing. Until housing conditions are bettered much of the work of the medical and nursing professions must be in vain. Until the mother can have adequate room in which to rear her family she will be merely disheartened by the advice she cannot follow and the ideals which she cannot attain.

INDEX

Printed in Great Britain by Hazell, Watson & Viney, Ld.,
London and Aylesbury.

Magazine of the London (Royal Free Hospital) School of
Medicine for Women Vol XXVI, No. 109, July 1931.

Physiognomy of Disease in Childhood.

*Being the Presidential Address delivered before the
Medical Society by* DR. CHODAK GREGORY,
on May 18th, 1931.

ALTHOUGH the vulgar use of the word Physiognomy is
generally applied to the face only, the original meaning
includes the art of judging by bodily form as well as facial
features, and may be taken in this instance to mean the art of
cultivating visual observation in our clinical examination of
patients.

I suppose the use of the eye is the first thing that most
clinicians impress upon students, yet it is strange how much
this use is neglected once the student's mind becomes absorbed
by the more difficult training of the ears and hands. So much
so that the untrained probationer nurse who is never taught
to use a stethoscope or palpate an abdomen can often put us
to shame by the direct and unfettered use of her eyes and
common-sense.

If inspection is useful in examination of the adult patient
whose facial expression may be masked by, on the one hand
rigorous self-control, or on the other, self-pity or even
malingering, how much more useful and reliable is the study
of childish expression which is rarely anything but genuine
and sincere. In infants especially, facial appearances may
have to replace history, for whereas in children of five years
and upwards there are always two histories to take into
account, that of the parent and that of the child himself, in
the case of infants only one history is available.

I should like to make it quite clear that I do not believe in
the "lightning diagnosis." Visual observation is only the
first part of an examination, and although in some cases it
must inevitably prejudice your final deductions it cannot
replace a full examination. It must at first be a conscious
study, a routine, taken in turn with the other methods of
examination and as systematically recorded ; but after a time
you will find yourselves practising it unconsciously and very
rapidly, so that a glance will imprint the picture on your
brain ; just as a society woman, without appearing to stare,
could let you have the minute details of her friend's costume,
though she has only passed her in the street.

Now, as to the method of observation, that must be done

with the greatest discretion and circumspection. Babies dislike being stared at almost as much as do animals. They generally prefer to do the staring themselves, and it is always advisable to ignore, or seem to ignore, a child for the first two minutes, to allow it time to take a good look at you and make up its mind about your character. If at the end of this time it has formed a low opinion of you, that is of course a pity, but it cannot be helped. This only applies to the ailing child; those who are very ill hardly mind whether you stare or not; and under those circumstances you may carry on your examination at leisure.

The child's facial expression may be hidden altogether if it screams or buries its head in the pillows ; but even screaming may be a useful sign—it at any rate gives the information that the lungs are not affected ; a screaming pneumonia is a contradiction in terms.

With so many examples of child physiognomy to draw from it is difficult to choose which to describe. All the more so as descriptions of facial expression, of general physique or of attitude must necessarily be somewhat fanciful, and because no two pædiatricians quite agree as to the interpretation of these observations.

I will select a few subjects and try to draw pictures of such appearances as have given me help at different times.

Taking first the acute diseases of childhood I would point out a very early sign in meningitis which is perhaps not enough emphasized in our text-books. That is, the stare ; not due, as in gastro-enteritis to depleted tissues, but due to early spasm of the eyelids. So equivocal are the other early signs and symptoms of meningitis, especially in infants, the vomiting, the constipation, the head retraction, that it is well to look out for this common phenomenon which has more than once drawn one's attention to the probable diagnosis. Once meningitis is well established the picture of muscular rigidity and ultimately opisthotonos is so obvious that none could mistake it, but by then a diagnosis is too late. In the later stages of meningeal rigidity, especially in tuberculous meningitis, the contraction of various facial muscles may give the baby what the late Dr. John Thomson described as " an air of deep thought and stern determination " very foreign to its tender age.

Another facial expression which is common to all ages is that of intense anxiety when the peritoneum has in any way lost its integrity. In a child with peritonitis, whether it be appendicular or pneumococcal or even a fulminating tuberculous infection, the mixture of suffering and anxiety on the face is very characteristic. There is often suffering and anxiety too in acute enteritis, but here the position and actions of the body will help to differentiate. The child in pain with enteritis (using this term in its widest sense) will toss about and often twist round, seeming to welcome the pressure of the bed on its abdomen. But with peritonitis its whole instinct is to keep still, lying on its back, legs drawn up to relax the abdominal muscles, diaphragm as motionless as a child's diaphragm can well be.

Allied to this peritonitic facial appearance is that of the infant suffering from hypertrophic pyloric stenosis. As far as one can tell he has no acute pain, but he rarely looks happy and he seems to be saying all the time, "There's something wrong in my inside. For heaven's sake do something about it."

Even the beginner could scarcely mistake the appearance of a child suffering from acute diffuse bronchiolitis or broncho-pneumonia. The noisy, laboured breathing, the cyanotic flush, the heaving chest, the recession of the lower thorax—altogether make an unequivocal picture which rarely deceives. Lobar pneumonia, on the other hand, is far more deceptive in its appearances. The respirations, though very rapid, may be so shallow as hardly to be perceptible, especially when pleurisy is present, while in other cases the lung condition may be entirely masked by a "cerebral" or "meningeal" onset. Look for the movement of the alae nasi, but at the same time bear in mind that children often use these nasal muscles in conditions other than pneumonia; they use them in the forced breathing of acidosis, and they use them sometimes from sheer apprehension, like a nervous horse. I have been asked what is the meaning of the one-sided flush which often appears on the cheek of a child suffering from pneumonia. Apart from conjecturing that the sympathetics on one side are stimulated and on the other are not, I do not know. What it does *not* tell us is which side we shall find the pneumonic patch. One important thing I would have you bear in mind. Be sure, when you see that there is respiratory distress, to ascertain what part of the respiratory passages is affected. I have seen acute obstruction from laryngeal diphtheria sent in to hospital as pneumonia, but there should be no mistaking the stridor of blocked larynx, once you have thought of the possibility.

Among colour schemes, the flush and cyanosis are most obvious, but look too for the dirty pallor of the toxic child, the greyness of collapse, the sub-icteric tinge of early jaundice, and in case of apparent anæmia, look especially at the lips— they are a surer guide than the skin.

Make yourself thoroughly familiar with the expression, as well as with the type of movement found in chorea. You may say chorea is easy to diagnose at sight. It generally is; but every now and then you will come across cases of multiple habit spasms or of irregular post-encephalitic movements which are very hard to differentiate from true chorea. You will then be glad to have studied the chorea face with its easy smile and quick tears and its extraordinary family resemblance to other choreas.

When we come to consider chronic disease there arises that vexed question whether or not there exists such a thing as a " diathesis " of disease, an inborn tendency; and if so, are the various diatheses marked by the possession of special facial and bodily features. The older physicians described in some detail two types of person who might have a predisposition to tuberculous disease; the " sanguine," with clear skin, pink and white complexion, silky hair and bright eyes; and the " phlegmatic " or scrofulous, the thickset child with coarse features and muddy complexion. Modern opinion has drifted away from these conceptions, and the French especially have tried to show that tuberculosis is purely an infectious disease and that no such thing as an hereditary diathesis exists. Nevertheless I think that most of us would be loath to give up the idea that a certain characteristic facial and bodily appearance can help us in the diagnosis of tuberculosis, though it is most important not to let such an appearance excuse a slovenly examination or over-influence our judgment.

The same questions arise with regard to rheumatism; the blonde child, fair, preferably red-haired, is looked upon with more suspicion when it complains of pains in its limbs than is the dark child, yet in a recent paper a medical officer at one of the L.C.C. Rheumatism hospitals showed that there was no such preponderance of fair-haired children among his many hundred rheumatism cases.

Another type of child that is frequently described is the

"lymphatic" or "pudding-faced" child, but the very existence of "lymphatism" has recently been called in doubt, so perhaps the less said about that the better.

Many children will be brought to you with vague general symptoms of ill-health, and you will see the very striking appearance of "dark marks under the eyes." This shadow is common and has been quoted as a part of many syndromes, such as chronic indigestion, acidosis, septic absorption, masturbation. I do not, for that reason, think it is in any way specific, it is only a general indication of lowered vitality; indeed some children exhibit the "dark marks" whenever they have undergone unusual physical or mental exertion.

There is one subject about which I believe you will very often be called upon to give an opinion, if your practice lies to any great extent among children, and that is the subject of mental deficiency in all its grades. When the suspicion first arises in the mother's mind that her baby is not quite normal she will bring it to you as to one who should be able to tell at sight. Sometimes she will bring it at two or three months old, sometimes it is surprisingly late before she has noticed any abnormality. I need not enter now into the details of examination in such case, except to mention the necessity of getting a very minute and careful history in the first place, but I should like to warn you that appearances may be most deceptive here. There are a few types of mental deficiency which can be literally diagnosed at a glance—the mongolian idiot, the microcephalic, the hydrocephalic and the cretin. But the simple primary amentias which form the greater bulk of all mentally deficients are not so obvious at first sight. The dull eye that one can never catch, the vacant expression, the grimace and bubbling at the mouth, are all suggestive, but it is important to remember that the squinting child with its mouth open has an extraordinarily stupid appearance, yet both squint and mouth-breathing may be explained on common physical grounds. Another point to remember about the seemingly backward child is that prolonged illness, debility, under-feeding and even isolation can hold back the development of the child's mind to such an extent that it may indeed appear to be hopelessly deficient, yet in reality its powers of normal development under improved circumstances are infinite. Be very cautious, therefore, about the diagnosis of mental deficiency from appearance; you will never be forgiven if you are proved to be wrong.

I will not quote any more instances of the physiognomy of disease because I no not wish to confuse you, but you will be constantly finding many more. Do not be content to take other people's descriptions, but use your own imaginations, and gradually the appearances of disease will become more and more familiar to you. You are not expected, unless you specialise in the subject, to recognise the rare abnormalities such as ocular hypertelorism, oxycephaly or acrocephalo-syndactylia, but you should have an acquaintance with the physiognomy of all common diseases. Never let the X-ray and the microscope take from you the use of your own eyes and never let the reading of books take from you the use of your own brains.

H. H. C. G.

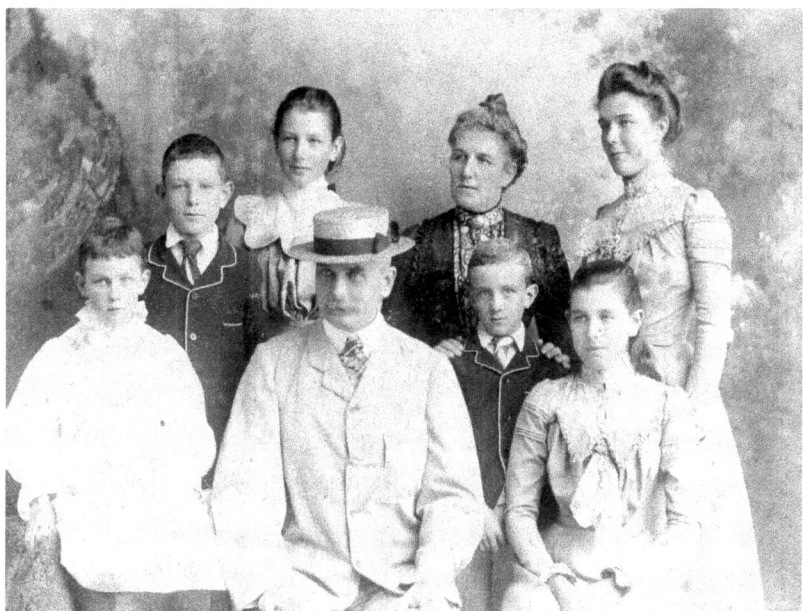

Figure 1 The Cuthbert Family

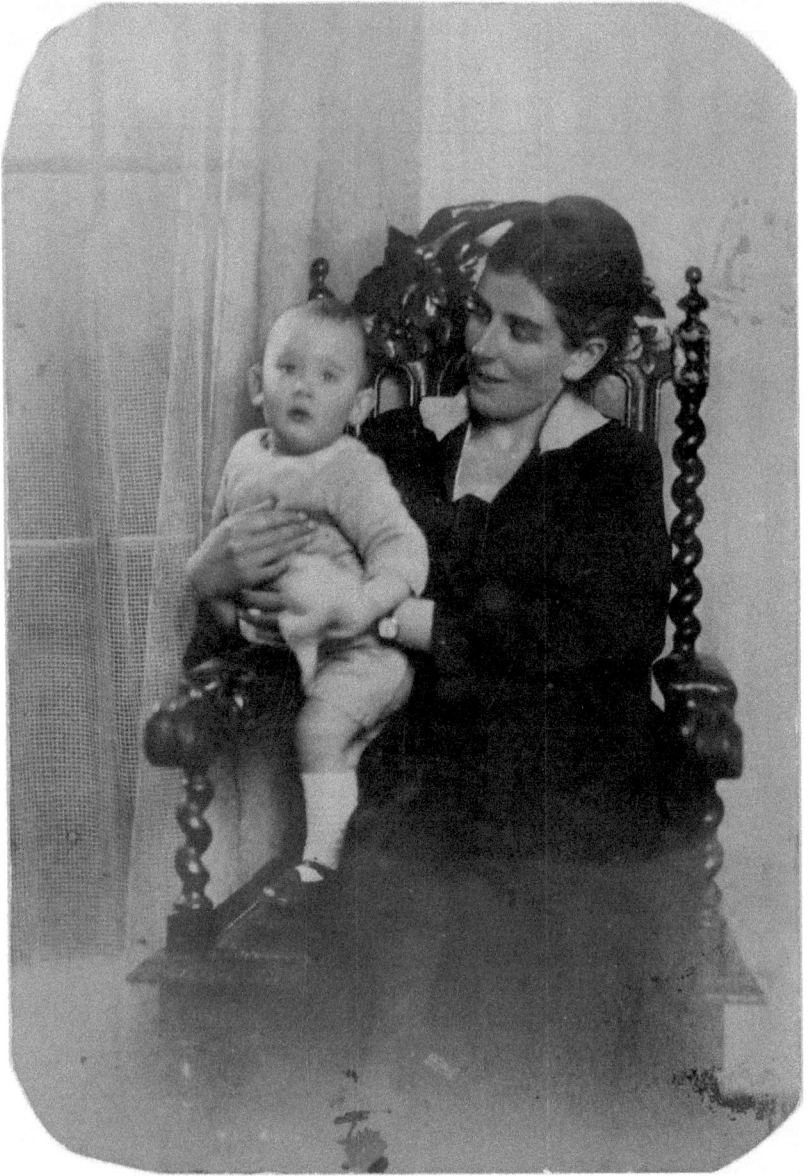

Figure 2 Hazel Chodak and Basil Gregory

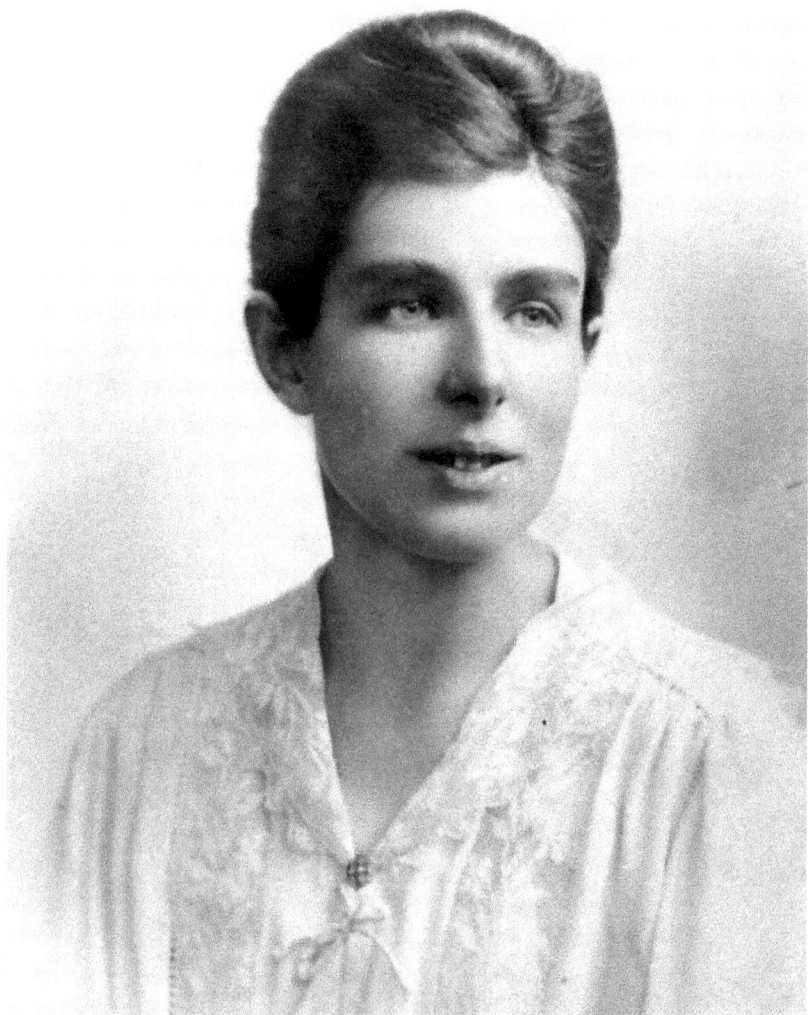

Figure 3 Hazel Chodak Gregory c. 1915

1898 – Houghton Grange, Huntingdon, Cambridgeshire

Home / Buildings / Architecture of England / Architecture of East England / Architecture of Cambridgeshire /

Architect: James Ransome

SEE ALSO

1898

Architecture of Cambridgeshire

country houses

Huntingdon

James Ransome

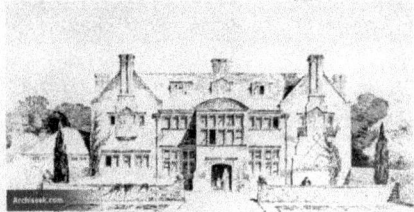

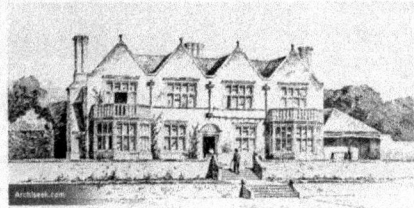

Houghton Grange has lain empty for over 25 years since the poultry research business who used it for decades along with rest of the estate closed. It is now in a bad way due to neglect and vandalism. There are two horrific 1960's laboratory extensions either side of the main house.

"Houghton Grange, now in course of completion for Mr. Harold Coote, is situated upon Houghton Hill, a few miles from Huntingdon, and commands an extensive view of the surrounding country. It is approached from the main road by a long straight avenue of limes on the north side, while to the south are the terraces, gardens, and lawn, leading down to the River Ouse. The house stands upon a roughly hammer-dressed base of Weldon stone, and has mullions and dressings of the same material, of which the carving has been executed by Mr. Henry Price, of Kensington. The walls are of red brick, and the roof hung with old green tiles. The plan is a plain parallelogram, whose only excrescences are the bay windows and chimneys, and, in addition to the accommodation shown, there are four bedrooms and a box-room on the second floor. The hall and drawing-room are panelled in oak, the former having above the panelling a frieze of red brickwork and an oak-framed ceiling. The rooms on the first floor are low, with the exception of the four principal bedrooms, which have barrel ceilings in the gables. A lodge has been built at the drive gates, and some of the old farm buildings are in process of conversion into stables. The drawing which we illustrate was shown at the Royal Academy this year. The architect is Mr. James Ransome, of London." Published in The Building News. December 9 1898.

Figure 4 Houghton Grange

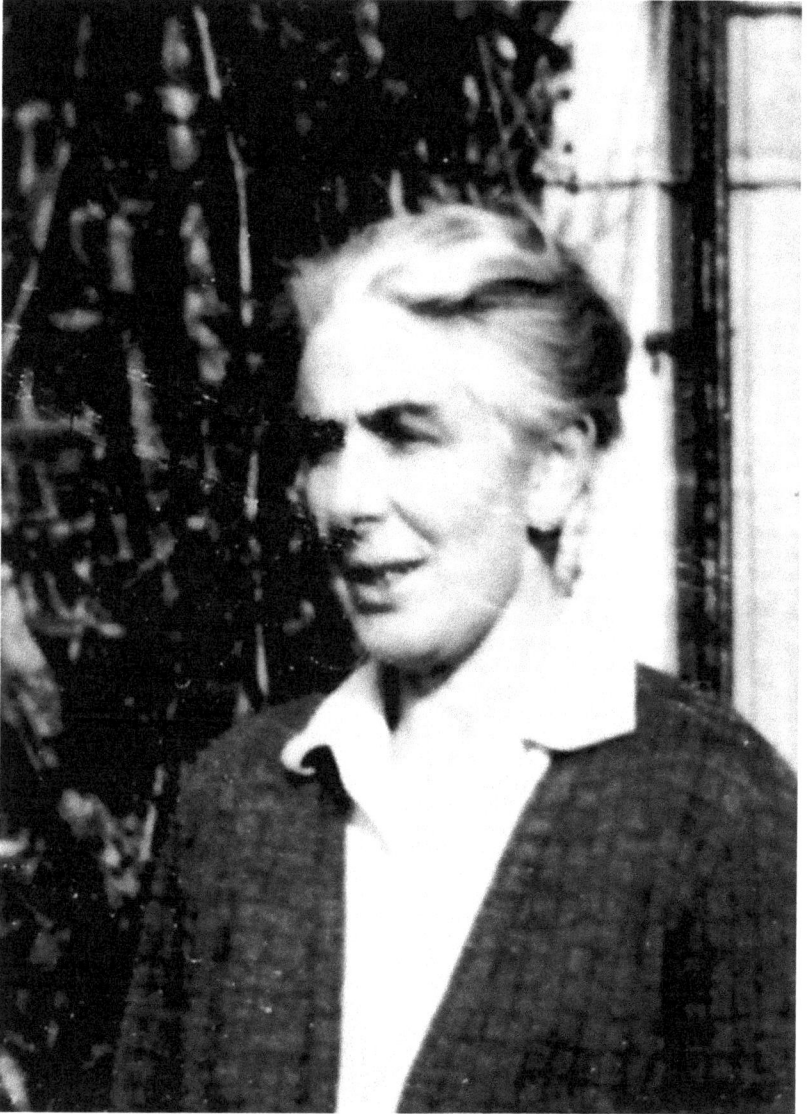

Figure 5 Hazel Chodak-Gregory in her 50s

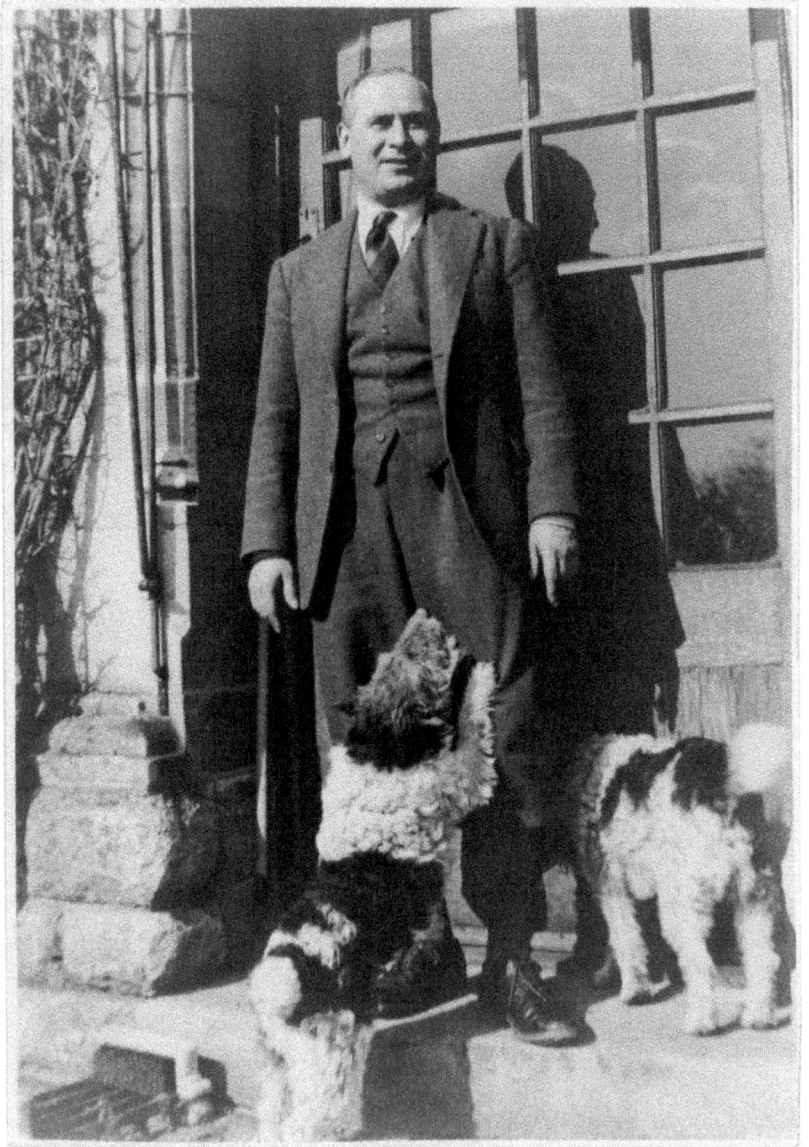

Figure 6 Dr Alexis Chodak-Gregory

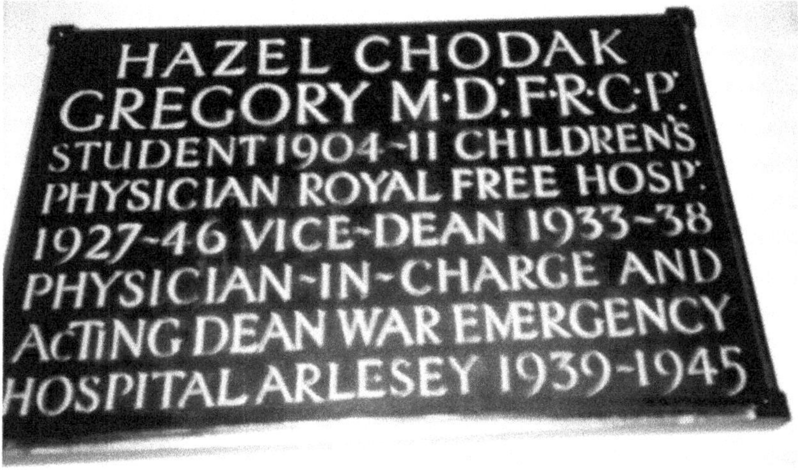

Figure 7 Royal Free Plaque to Hazel Chodak-Gregory

For Product Safety Concerns and Information please contact our EU representative GPSR@taylorandfrancis.com
Taylor & Francis Verlag GmbH, Kaufingerstraße 24, 80331 München, Germany